MW01291364

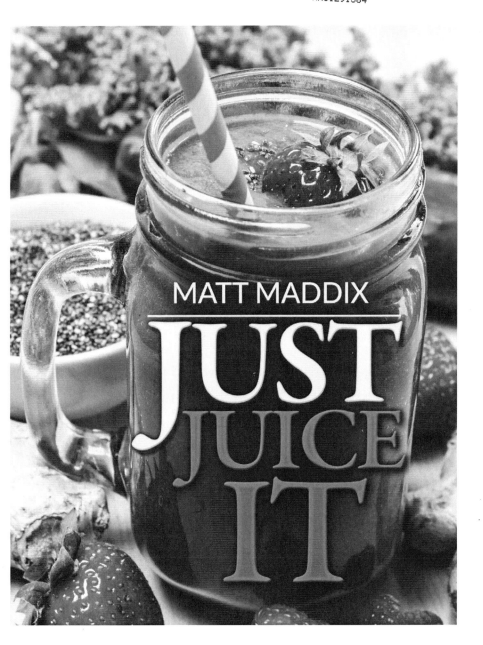

MATT MADDIX

JUST JUICE IT

Just Juice It!
By Matt Maddix

Table of Contents

Foreword

In his second book on Juicing, Matthew J. Maddix, author of "Just Juice It," writes with passion and energy, and the information he has gleaned from his own experiences are reflected in the book! He is very radical in his belief that juicing is packed with great nutritional value and is brimming over with the essential fluids of life! He has discovered that the JUICE of fresh fruits and vegetables is the richest available source of vitamins, minerals and enzymes, and that raw juice becomes Fuel for the body by enabling it to easily assimilate those valuable nutrients!

Someone once wrote: "Our medicine is all around us. Our food is our pharmacy. Herbs are our medicine. The oceans are our healers." Matt has made this believable!

It's been said, "The Greatest Wealth is Health!" Matt Maddix is working hard to bring "wealth" to those who suffer with any kind of disease or sickness! This book will enrich, enlighten, inform, and provide the "how to" about the miracle of juicing! It is written so that even a beginner can understand it. Good healthy juicing should be your medicine instead of man-made drugs. Juicing helps you to start feeling better and will help to keep you well!

Matt discusses subjects such as: Health benefits of juicing, How to live a healthy lifestyle, Foods that fight cancer, Advice for overweight people, and a section of Questions and Answers. Your life will be changed if the principles taught in this book are applied. God has given Matt the ability to inspire people, and as you read this book, you will be inspired, challenged, and motivated to go forward and embrace a healthier lifestyle.

Joy Haney
Author, Speaker

Chapter 1

Why I started Juicing and Eating Healthy

I had a wake-up call when one of my friends died suddenly of a heart attack, leaving behind his wife and kids. Who would have expected a man to die so young? It was very sobering; his wife, family and friends suffered greatly over this loss. It broke my heart and was a wake-up call for me to take my health seriously. I remember standing at his funeral and feeling very frustrated as they had to pull his daughter away from the casket. I thought to myself, "He didn't have to die!" There is a scripture in Ecclesiastes 7:17 that says, "Why be foolish and die before your time?" Although we all have a time to go, we need to honor God by taking care of our body. Because I've seen so many people suffering with ill health, I have made up my mind to live every single day with the purpose of doing the best I can to live a healthy lifestyle. I truly get so sick and tired of always seeing people sick. Our country is consumed with sickness sand disease. We can lay much of the blame the food industry for this. We live in a GMO, fast food, and highly processed food world. We rarely eat home-cooked, nutritional meals at home. It's so sad to me that many homes never juice or eat raw fruits and vegetables. I'm am very driven and feel so much passion to tell my story and get this book in the hands of people. I want our children to fall in love with juicing. There is no reason that juicing can't become a family affair and the norm in every household. Juicing is life! Juicing is a blast! We can't live without it.

My eyes have really been opened over the years as I have traveled across the country and have seen so many people tired, sick, lethargic, and struggling to give 100% to God, family and their dreams. In those early days of my travels, I was eating cheeseburgers, fries, and pizza, while drinking white mochas from Starbucks, Mountain Dews, and Cokes. Although I owned a juicer, I rarely used it. Instead, I drank the beverages that contained only 5% real juice. I was also out of shape, had put on 40 lbs. of extra weight and was not in optimal health. I felt horrible, tired, depressed and was always getting sick.

I just took a break from writing and pulled out my Nutri-Bullet and filled it with Spinach, Watermelon, Pineapple, Raspberries and Grapes and filled it with cold water, blended it all together and drank it. It makes me feel so refreshed, invigorated, and alive. I've become addicted to juicing as I have learned more about the health benefits of juicing on a daily basis.

I would strongly recommend that you get into the habit of juicing at least two-three times per day. I can tell a big difference in my life when I don't juice. For those of you who don't think you can juice or you think juicing is nasty, just try it for a few weeks. Your body will become accustomed to it and will begin to crave it. Just stick with the process, and in time, you'll see massive results from juicing on a daily basis. My whole entire life is different because of juicing. I'm never sick, always feel extreme high energy, experience amazing, restful sleep at night, no aches or pains in my body, not to mention the great feeling of being skinny and in shape.

My first meal of the day includes a big breakfast, which usually consists of oatmeal with almond milk, a spoonful of coconut oil, blueberries, raspberries, strawberries and almonds. Never skip breakfast! It is the most important meal of the day. After studying the habits of highly healthy people, I've learned that many of them eat every two-three hours. I've adopted this same mentality and usually will begin with my first juice two hours after eating my oatmeal. My first juice is the fruit drink mentioned above.

God expects us to make healthy choices in feeding and nourishing the body He has given us. For lunch, I eat a salad with turkey, balsamic vinaigrette, olive oil and some organic spinach leaves. It's one of my favorite meals of the day. You can add chicken and salmon to your salad if you are not a fan of turkey. After about two to three hours, it's time for my second juice of the day. My second juice is usually a straight up vegetable juice consisting of kale, celery, spinach, red bell pepper, tomatoes, water and garlic.

Yikes! Garlic, you say? Let me explain some of the healing powers of garlic. Garlic is truly a miracle plant. Through the ages, garlic has been known to kill cancers, fight against typhoid fever and dysentery, and disinfect, heal and strengthen battle wounds when there was a shortage of sulfur. Garlic has been shown in double-blind studies to reduce incidences of colon-rectal cancer, stomach cancer, breast cancer, etc. It is an anti-bacterial fighter against all foreign invaders to a healthy body. Garlic is famous for its healing power upon heart disease, which is the #1 cause of death in the United States today. This year alone, over one million people will die from it. 99% of all these heart attacks are caused by cholesterol and saturated fats blocking the coronary arteries. One research study revealed that countries where people had a high consumption of garlic, the incidence of heart disease was much lower than average. Garlic has been shown to lower serum cholesterol and triglyceride levels and reduce the build-up of atherosclerotic plaque in our arteries. High blood pressure has become a worldwide epidemic. Garlic has proven conclusively to reduce hypertension. Because of its powerful effect on blood pressure, the Japanese Food and Drug Administration has approved and listed garlic as an official drug in the Japanese pharmacopoeia. Many other studies have shown ways in which the miracle plant from God helps us on so many levels.

For dinner, my favorite meat is fish. One wish of mine is that people would start eating more white meat such as fish, turkey and chicken. It is best to eat wild caught fish rather than farmed and free-range poultry. Add some broccoli to that and you have a perfect meal. You can sauté broccoli with a little coconut or olive oil and add some spices, and it tastes delicious. Remember, if you are eating and juicing every two to three hours, you'll not feel as hungry and will actually lose weight by following this type of lifestyle.

I am very careful about eating white sugar or white flour because the fiber has been removed, depleting the body of vitamins and minerals, and causing a constipating effect. Rarely do I allow myself to eat red meat and fast food because they are known to cause health problems in the body. Why choose nutritionally depleted foods when you can have better foods that not only satisfy your hunger, but also taste delicious because you are receiving a higher level of nutrition?

I challenge you to eat a healthy salad everyday that is not loaded with cheeses and the wrong kind of dressings. Since God gave us life and a purpose while we are alive on this earth, we need to make the best choices that are available to us so we can fulfill that purpose. Juicing and eating right will give you massive energy and help you feel great about your body.

The goal of this book is to challenge you to commit to a higher standard of living by changing your lifestyle and the way you eat. I don't like the word diet because diets are temporary, but lifestyle changes can be a forever thing.

If you think about it for a moment, nutrition isn't the alternative system. Drugs are the alternative system, and they are far from natural. Drugs are really a patching-up system of medicine, a Band-Aid. At best, drugs are a short-term method that can arrest a harmful organism and stabilize body systems to the point where your own individual immune system can take over and reestablish health.

God made the body to heal itself. If we will do our best to feed the body the proper nutrients and feed our mind the proper thoughts, we will live a healthier life than if we feed on things that have been proven to cause health problems in the body.

We must take a measure of responsibility for our health, for no one has more access to us than we ourselves. The question we should ask before putting something our body is, "How will this enhance my health? Will it cause disease or will it bring vital health, energy, or cure?" I am a weight loss coach and have helped people lose over 100 pounds the healthy way by changing their habits and lifestyle. One of the things that I have them do is slow down and get into the habit of asking these seven questions before they eat:

1. *Is it Healthy?*
2. *How will it make me feel 30 minutes after eating it?*
3. *Is there a Healthier option?*
4. *Why do I want to eat this?*
5. *Will this cause me to gain weight?*
6. *Will I regret eating this?*
7. *Would a fit and healthy person eat this?*

Most of my clients that do really well and lose the weight follow my challenge of eating every two to three hours and juicing at least twice per day as a lifestyle and not a diet. Therefore, even after the inspiration from reading this book wears off, you'll change your lifestyle to the point that you are in the habit of juicing everyday so that you'll still be juicing for the rest of your life.

I started juicing because I value my life and love my 12-year-old son more than anything on earth. I plan on living a long, healthy and high quality life. I'm not going to cheat my son and family by neglecting my health and living like a slob. Our families deserve more! I want to be the type of dad that has energy to play with my son and do things with him. I want to set the example of health for him and make sure that I teach him the right habits.

Turn juicing into an adventure and let children help make their own juices. Children who might be fussy about eating fruits or vegetables can be encouraged to drink a glass of juice that they have helped prepare. My son started juicing at a very young age and used to love helping me juice. Caleb literally requests juice on a daily basis because his body can feel the difference from when he juices and when he doesn't. If you are a parent reading this book, I strongly encourage you to start a juicing routine for your kids at a young age and condition their bodies and minds to drinking one to three juices per day. I strongly encourage husbands and wives to do this together as a couple. Husbands, don't let your wife be the only one taking her health and body seriously. Too many men let themselves go and expect their wives to look like Hollywood super models while they continue to turn into fat slobs. Men, take the lead and show your wife and kids that you are serious about your health. Real men juice!

Obesity is becoming a major problem in America. Not just among adults, but also among our children. Our country is the most obese country in the world. Something must change, and it starts by making the commitment to return back to fruits and vegetables. We must change the way we eat and live our lives. We are literally killing ourselves. We are living a sluggish, lazy, sick and short-lived life because we are not filling our bodies with the nutrients that it needs. We must become fanatics about juicing. We have to get tough about it. Nobody will become a healthy and a regular juicer until they get determined and make up their mind that they are going to be healthy. Was it easy for me at first? Yes it was, because I went all in and threw away ALL the junk in my home. I stopped drinking all soda, started drinking water and juiced two to three times a day. I literally started to LOVE juicing. I loved the process of taking the juicer out of the cabinet, the noise of my juicer and the very process of even cleaning it. It was so energizing, exciting and invigorating. The fact that I always feel so good and have such energy to live the life of my dreams, do you think that I'm going to worry about how "long it takes" to juice or clean up the juicer? No! It became easy for me because I stopped whining about it and decided to refuse to say one negative or sarcastic word about juicing or the process of juicing. Too many of us don't take our health seriously. We play too many games and take such a passive approach about it.

I'm extremely excited about you getting started into juicing and making it your lifestyle. Although you may have thought that juicing was too time-consuming or distasteful, in time it will become an enjoyable daily routine for you and your family.

Chapter 2

The Health Benefits of Juicing

The health benefits of juicing are enormous, and it's such an easy way to consume our "five-a-day" servings of fruits and vegetables that even children can be encouraged to drink juice without a fuss.

One of the benefits of juicing is that approximately 95% of the food value of the fruit or vegetable is released instantly into your bloodstream, thus bypassing the time-consuming digestive process. Fresh fruit and vegetable juices contain the purest natural form of concentrated vitamins, minerals, antioxidants, and enzymes that work together in cleansing, alkalizing, and balancing the body as it detoxifies all your cells and organs by stimulating them to eliminate toxic waste, which promotes healing and restoration of energy and vitality.

One glass of juice can contain more than one fruit or vegetable; in fact, it can contain a variety, making it colorful, balanced and healthy. Juicing one apple and two carrots would qualify as two of your "five-a-day." Fresh fruit and vegetable juices speed up the ability of your white blood cells to cleanse your blood and tissues of bacteria, virus, fungus, and many harmful pathogenic microorganisms such as tumors and malignant cancer cells. No disease can live in a healthy, pure environment, so by putting mineral rich juices into your body, you become cleaner, healthier and more energetic.

A nutritious, tall glass of fruit or vegetable juice can replace your breakfast or lunch. A glass of fresh juice gives you sufficient goodness and energy to keep you going, and has more nutrition than six bowls of assorted fruits and vegetables. For example, it would be difficult to eat a pound of carrots, but making ten and a half ounces of carrot juice from that pound of carrots provides instantly absorbable vitamins, minerals, and trace elements that are so vital for your well-being.

The basic key to nourishing your body comes from the life of those intangible elements in your food, known as enzymes. The elements which enable the body to be nourished and to live are the enzymes which cause seeds to sprout and plants to grow. Enzymes have been described as complex substances, which enable us to digest food and absorb it into our blood. It has been claimed that Enzymes digest cancers. Enzymes are catalysts, and as such, they promote action or change without altering or changing their own status. With this brief explanation, you are better able to appreciate the value, reason, and logic of choosing the food with which you intend to nourish your body. Raw fruits and vegetables are full of enzymes which nourish the cells and tissues of your body in the fastest and most efficient manner possible.

Some people ask, why not just eat the fruit and vegetables instead of juicing and drinking them? Solid food requires many hours of digestive activity before its nourishment is finally available to the cells and tissues of the body, while juices are very quickly digested and assimilated, sometimes in a matter of minutes, with a minimum of effort on the part of the digestive system. Of course you should eat fruits and vegetables in addition to your juicing. Juicing is like a blood transfusion in that it goes immediately into the blood, requiring hardly any time for digesting.

Juicing can absolutely change your life by helping you regain your health, lose weight, and increase energy. You'll sleep better, feel better, and enjoy life more when you become a daily juicer. It's worth the time and money to ensure that you live a healthy and feel-good life. Below is a list of the top ten benefits of juicing; they are in no certain order.

1. *Weight loss*
2. *Healthy and fit body*
3. *Fight cancer and disease*
4. *Give you more energy*
5. *Help you feel better in your body*
6. *Cleansing and Detoxification*
7. *Antioxidants*
8. *Alkalinity*
9. *Hydration*
10. *Better Nutrient Absorption*

So as you can see, juicing is extremely beneficial for you. I'm sure that by now you are a believer in the power of juicing. The days of making excuses and procrastinating are over. It's time for you to stop waiting. Today is the day for you to make up your mind to get focused on your health. Yes, right now as you read this book, I want you to see that juicing is for you and that it will completely revolutionize your health, body, mind and spirit. You'll become a happier, more fulfilled, energetic, enthusiastic, active and more passionate human being when you start juicing. You'll not have to live in fear of sickness or disease anymore. Juicing will give you a peace of mind about your Health. I'm convinced that juicing can conquer any sickness and disease. If I came down with an illness, I would literally eliminate any stress, negative emotions, worry, fear, guilt or bitterness from my life. I would stop eating all red meat, sugars, and processed foods and do nothing but juice and eat organic white meat. Of course, I strongly urge you to consult with your doctor. I'm only sharing what I would do because I believe in the benefits of juicing so much that I believe juicing can cure most sickness and diseases, especially if all negative emotions and stress were eliminated from your life. Therefore, that is why I already do all of this in my life now as a lifestyle because I'm more into prevention rather than cure. I've learned that if you live, eat and juice as if you were sick or struck with disease, then it's almost 100% certain that you'll live a very healthy life free of sickness and disease.

The Benefit of Carrot Juice

Carrot juice has the effect of helping to normalize the entire system. It is the richest source of Vitamin A which the body can quickly assimilate and also contains an ample supply of Vitamins B, C, D, E, G and K. It is a valuable aid in the improvement and maintenance of the bone structure of the teeth. Raw Carrot juice is a natural solvent for ulcerous and cancerous conditions. It is a resistant to infections, doing its most efficient work in conjunction with the adrenal glands. It helps prevent infections of the eyes and throat as well as the respiratory organs. It also protects the nervous system and is unequalled for increasing vigor and vitality. It can give the skin a stain-like appearance, and is a great help in detoxifying the liver. Raw Carrot juice is very rich in the vital organic alkaline elements of sodium and potassium. It also contains a good supply of calcium, magnesium, and iron.

It is interesting that the people, who live solely on fresh raw foods supplemented with a sufficient volume and variety of fresh raw vegetable and fruit juices, do not develop cancers.

The Benefit of Green Juices

Green juices are healing, stabilizing and calming. It took me a little getting used to. However, I have fallen in love with drinking green juice. If you want a quick pick-me-up, drink carrot juice. But for long-term energy, take a green drink. If you are exhausted, restless, or feeling scattered, drink green.

A green juice is not just a blood cleanser; it is a nerve tonic, which alkalizes and mineralizes. Chlorophyll is the chemical formed by the chloroplast cells of green plants. Without chlorophyll, all animal life on earth would become extinct. Amazingly, this "blood of plants" is structurally similar to hemin, the protein portion of hemoglobin that carries oxygen. Green plants, whether they are wheatgrass, kale, or broccoli, get their energy from the sun. Photons of light from the sunshine are captured in the cells of green plants called chloroplasts. As the chloroplasts absorb the light, their electrons become excited; they literally dance in the sunshine. The energy they are charged with is stored (like batteries) as ATP. The ATP then reduces carbon dioxide and water to oxygen and carbohydrates. The oxygen exits the leaf and fills the atmosphere with fresh air. The carbohydrates remain as food. Both the oxygen and carbohydrates become the basic sustenance for animal life. If chemists were able to duplicate photosynthesis by artificial means, we would have an endless source of power – solar energy.

You'll be seeing some of my favorite green drink recipes in this book. I've seen first-hand the benefits of drinking greens and how much energy it gives me day in and day out. This is the cleansing energy that goes into your body when you drink green juices.

In conjunction with drinking green juices, one of my daily habits is to drink 2-4 ounces of wheat grass. Always try to drink wheat grass on an empty stomach and wait 30 minutes before eating anything solid. I personally couldn't stand drinking Wheat Grass at first. It made me gag. However, like they say, "You don't feel your way into action, you act your way into feeling." I knew that it was good for me, and I made myself do it even when I had to plug my noise at times. My son Caleb almost threw up the first few times that he drank Wheat Grass. However, the good news is that both of us have adjusted and now we can slam 4-6 ounces without even needing a chaser. I strongly recommend that you drink it straight from the actual Wheat Grass plan rather than through a pill or powder form. You'll get more nutritional value from drinking it from the actual grass.

I'm a fanatic about Wheat Grass and am a believer in the nutritional value that you get from drinking it. I've watched Wheat Grass take away joint muscle pain and help heal sickness and disease. Wheat Grass contains over 100 elements needed by man. If grown in organic soil, it absorbs 92 of the 115 minerals from the soil.

Wheatgrass has a strong cleansing effect on the digestive tract. Here are the top 20 benefits of wheat grass.

Benefits of Drinking Wheat Grass

1. *Purifies and rebuilds blood*
2. *Cleanses the colon*
3. *Alkalizes the blood*
4. *Purges the Liver*
5. *Neutralizes toxins*
6. *Oxygenates Cells*
7. *Heals wounds*
8. *Detoxifies cellular fluids*
9. *Heals intestinal walls*
10. *Raises enzyme activity*
11. *Beneficial to the treatment of skin disease*
12. *Improves blood sugar problems*
13. *Helps prevent tooth decay*
14. *Is Gluten-free because it's cut before grain forms*
15. *Increases energy, strength and endurance*
16. *Suppresses appetite*
17. *Treats arthritis*
18. *Reduces fatigue*
19. *Gets rid of bad breath and body odor*
20. *Clears sinus congestion*

Fact: "Drinking 2 ounces of Wheat Grass is equivalent to eating 5 pounds of raw vegetables."

Hopefully by now you are ready to start drinking Wheat Grass on a daily basis. I recommend at least 2 ounces per day. People often say, "It's too expensive to drink Wheat Grass and juice!" Friends, you haven't even seen expensive until you see the price of sickness and disease. I'd do whatever it takes, live without cable and almost anything else before I would stop juicing and drinking Wheat Grass. I'd rather go without furniture, eating out or vacations before I gave up my Wheat Grass and juicing. Just be willing to do whatever it takes. There is something about it. When you make the commitment, it has such an effect on your life that it even carries over and causes you to earn and make more money. When you honor God by taking excellent care of your health, He has a way of providing the means for you to juice and take care of yourself. You'll never regret investing in your health. I've found that over a long period of time, eating right and juicing actually saves me money. My best advice is that you keep a very enthusiastic positive and abundant attitude and mentality toward health, juicing and exercise.

Chapter 3

How to Live a Healthy Lifestyle

I've been blessed to be around some of the healthiest people in the world, and I've learned that they are no different than you and I. Most of these healthy people love pizza, ice cream, cake and a good cheeseburger like the rest of us. Most of the healthy people that I know have real struggles, temptations and food cravings like the rest of us. They are normal human beings that have learned some secrets of healthy living. The only difference is that they live a healthy lifestyle by having healthy habits. I've learned that it all comes down to our habits. It's like what I teach my Weight Loss Coaching clients: you can lose the weight, live a healthy life, and be skinny without dieting and depriving yourself of food. You just need to learn how to live a Healthy Life. I'm going to show you in this chapter how to live a healthy lifestyle.

1. Healthy Attitude and Emotions

The first thing that I work on with my clients is changing their attitude. I've worked with a lot of obese people, and the first thing that I notice about them is that many of them have a very depressed, negative and bad attitude. I truly believe that attitude is everything. The first step toward having a healthy attitude is eliminating all bitterness and unforgiveness from your life. I believe that most sickness and disease is a result of bitterness and stress. I'm convinced that negative emotions actually bring sickness to our bodies. I want you to let go of the past and stop allowing the pain of yesterday to sabotage your joy, peace of mind and most importantly, your health. Carrying bitterness toward people that hurt you isn't worth cancer or death. I've watched people actually get sick because they held grudges, bitterness and hate toward people who hurt them. I once had major pain in my knee when I was in an unhealthy, toxic

21

relationship. The second I ended the relationship, the sharp pain in my knee went away immediately. It's amazing how much negative emotions are connected to our bodies.

Unhealthy Emotions to Eliminate:

1. *Bitterness*
2. *Complaining*
3. *Negativity*
4. *Anger*
5. *Resentment*
6. *Guilt*
7. *Shame*
8. *Fear*
9. *Doubt*
10. *Stress*
11. *Anxiety*
12. *Depression*
13. *Loneliness*
14. *Insecurity*
15. *Worry*

These types of emotions will cause illness and weaken our immune system. Not to mention that they will also cause such major energy loss in our life. It's not worth carrying this extra baggage. We must take it all to God in prayer and make up our mind not to allow any negative and toxic emotions to rule in our mind and heart. God is able to heal us from all this toxic emotional baggage so that we can live a healthy, vibrant, energetic, happy and fulfilled life.

Yes, positive thinking and gratitude will completely change your attitude. In fact, if you would practice being more grateful, you would see a major change in your energy. Living a healthy lifestyle will give you good energy and living with good energy is so good for your family, friends and loved ones. In fact, living a healthy life can change the vibe and energy of our homes to the degree that our kids actually love being home. Many of our kids are not even at peace in their own homes because many parents are living with negative attitudes and emotions. Parents, for the sake of your children, get healthy. Your kids need you to be enthusiastic, happy, energetic and vibrant. Get rid of the depression, anger, bitterness, hate and resentment. Proverbs 17:22 says, "A merry heart does good like medicine!" We need happiness and joy back in our lives. The secret to living a super happy life is found in maintaining the right attitude and healthy emotions.

Set the example and determine the mood of your home by living with a great attitude. I'm convinced that one of the reasons why my son Caleb is so confident as a young boy is because of the attitude of joy, happiness and peace that I've displayed in front of him. Our kids need to see a lot of laughter and happiness from their parents.

2. Get into the Habit of Daily Exercise

Walking is good medicine. Cardiologists say that good physical exercise is prevention for heart disease. When we walk, the muscles take over their proper share of the work. Circulation speeds up, and the heart rate and blood pressure go down. I'm convinced that anyone can become healthy by doing daily physical fitness. One of the signs of a healthy person is that they do some form of exercise everyday. Of the 30 people that I have personally coached to lose weight through my personal one on one weight loss coaching system, all of them hadn't exercised for years when I first started coaching with them. See, it's really not that hard. Those that are healthy tend to exercise daily and those that are not healthy, don't. Friends, you can no longer make excuses about this. Daily exercise is a must if you want to be healthy. Is it easy? Well, it depends on how you approach it and what kind of priority you place it in

your life. I'm of the opinion that skipping exercise is not an option whatsoever. In fact, it's one of the most important aspects of your life.

Most people want to live a long life. Therefore, we should do the things that healthy people do. Not only do I want to live a long life, but I also want to live a long, healthy, disease-free life. Because I refuse to die young and allow disease to destroy my health, I'm very passionate about getting in at least 30 minutes of intense cardio everyday.

There are many different types of cardio that you can do. Here is a list of the top 10 cardio exercises that I've found to produce results and get the body moving:

1. *Walking*
2. *Jogging*
3. *Biking*
4. *Swimming*
5. *Aerobic Dance*
6. *Basketball*
7. *Rollerblading*
8. *Elliptical*
9. *Rowing*
10. *Hiking*

I personally mix these 10 exercises up and do a combination of several. You choose the type of exercises that you enjoy doing so long as you get your body moving. Many have a passive and negative attitude about exercise. Friends, it's all a matter of attitude and priority. When you start thinking positive and upbeat about exercise, you'll have more energy and passion to want to do it. I'm very strict with my clients that they exercise at least 30 minutes everyday. Many of them hated it at first, but all of them eventually fell in love with it, and their body started to crave more of it. Physical exercise stimulates various brain chemicals that leave you feeling happier and more relaxed. You'll find many benefits of exercise. Here are a few of them that should motivate and inspire you to do it:

1. *Controls weight gain*
2. *Improves the mood*
3. *Boosts energy*
4. *Promotes better sleep*
5. *Puts the spark back in your sex life*
6. *Reduces stress*
7. *Improves self confidence*
8. *Alleviates anxiety*
9. *Boosts brainpower*
10. *Helps control addictions*
11. *Increases creativity*
12. *Clears the mind*
13. *Improves body image*

Physical exercise can be a fun way to spend some time with your family, spouse, kids and friends. It gives you a chance to unwind, enjoy the outdoors or simply engage in activities that make you happy. Want to feel better, have more energy and perhaps even live longer? Look no further than exercise. Friends, exercise is the single best thing you can do for your brain in terms of mood, memory and learning.

3. Get plenty of rest –

God actually created our bodies to need rest. I do this daily internet talk show with my business partner, Mike Hopkins, and in our show this week we talked about, "The hardest Spiritual lesson that I had to learn and why." For me the hardest lesson to learn was that my body needed to rest. I literally have the kind of mental toughness and energy that could go without much sleep at all. I can function with two to three hours of sleep per night. It's not always easy to turn off your passion and make your body rest when you feel so good all the time. For example, it's 11:34 pm as I write this chapter. I've been writing since 9 pm, and I haven't moved. I'm having a blast doing this, and I want to keep on going. However, I still have this little voice in the back of my mind reminding me that I need to rest my body and get a good night's rest. Easier said than done right? For sure!

I actually had to learn this the hard way, my friends. I found myself literally on my deathbed in Canada a few years ago. I had a stress reaction that caused my throat to close up to the point where I could barely breathe. My Papa Rick (great man in my life that I've adopted to be my Papa) took me to the emergency room, and the doctor told us, "If you had waited 30 more minutes, you'd be dead!"

It was the wake-up call that shook me to my core. Hey doc, are you serious? No joke? Really? I was literally 30 minutes from death? We are talking like, DEATH!

He said, "Maybe 30 minutes, but most likely 15!"

All because I had neglected the laws of health and violated God's plan for my body to rest. I was going 24/7 and felt justified because I was exercising and juicing and changing the world. Right? No! WRONG! I still needed to rest and get a good night's sleep every night if I was going to live a healthy lifestyle! I'll never forget that experience as long as I live. It was the most sobering moment of my life. I had been through a lot of stress and had been traveling so much. I felt great in my body, but knew I was run down. I knew that something wasn't right. I got on a plane to Canada and when I landed, I was having a hard time breathing and could feel my throat swelling. It was weird. I had never experienced anything like that before. However, I just thought it would go away. It didn't, and thank God that Papa Rick insisted that I go to the emergency room. I would have never gone, and the doctor told me that 15 minutes more of a delay would have been fatal. What's the lesson learned from this experience? Whew! Pretty emotional to write about this! I had forgotten until I started sharing! Well, I learned to slow down and love my family in the most loving, affectionate and passionate way. I also learned that none of us are actually Superman. We really do need to rest our body and take time to pull away from stress and the pressures of life. Sleep, relaxing, days off and regular vacations are actually good for our body.

I've actually learned how to sleep well and rest my body from stress. Here are the secrets to proper rest, relaxation and stress-free living:

1. *Go to bed before 11*
2. *Turn off your phone*
3. *Don't look at any media an hour before bed*
4. *No caffeine or alcohol 4 hours before bed*
5. *Drink some Chamomile tea before bed*
6. *Turn off the lights and turn on some candles*
7. *Write your To Do list for the next day*
8. *Meditate*
9. *Take naps*
10. *Wake up in a good mood*
11. *Exercise*
12. *Think positive and be grateful*
13. *Laugh*
14. *Walk the beach*
15. *Enjoy nature*
16. *Be with family and friends*
17. *Think positive thoughts*
18. *Pray and Connect with God*
19. *Create a bedtime ritual and routine*
20. *Have more fun and enjoy life*
21. *Visualize your dreams and future*

These are just some of the things that have really helped me live stress-free and actually get a good night's sleep. It's not just the sleep that matters; it's also the stress-free living that comes through doing the things that I mentioned and really living a Healthy lifestyle.

4. Laugh and Have Fun

Yes, laughing is actually a very important aspect of living a healthy life. I know people who never laugh and enjoy life and usually as a result, they are often sick, unhappy and full of misery. One thing you'll find as you study the life of the healthy is that many of them are lighthearted and have learned the healing power of laughing and having fun. Why take life so seriously and allow so much stress in your life? It actually sabotages your health and energy. You would see such a change in your body if you started laughing more and enjoying life the way you're supposed to enjoy it. Life is good! It's okay to have fun and laugh!

Too many people allow the stress of life and the issues of the past to keep them from having fun. I know people, who have lost loved ones, have grown up poor, or had it rough as a kid, and they feel guilty for having fun. God intended for us to have fun and enjoy His blessings on our life. The Bible actually tells that, "Laughter is like medicine to the soul!" I've known people who had a major disease in their life, and one of the reasons that they cured the sickness and disease was because they refused to allow stress in their life, and they started having fun and laughing on a daily basis. Try it! Your spouse, friends, employees and children will enjoy being around you more because you know how to have a good sense of humor and have fun. Here are some ideas that could help you have more laughter and playfulness in your life:

1. *Reminisce with old friends*
2. *Watch your favorite comedy*
3. *Play with Children*
4. *Visit an amusement park*
5. *Play games that make you laugh*
6. *Try something new*
7. *Spend time with fun people*
8. *Listen to a fun song from your childhood*
9. *Play in a bouncy house – Jumping with kids is fun*
10. *Share funny jokes and stories with friends*
11. *Build a sand castle*
12. *Go for a hike*
13. *Visit the beach*
14. *Play with animals*
15. *Play with toys* ☺
16. *Dance, yes do it*
17. *Play in the rain*
18. *Laugh at yourself*
19. *Play funny board games*
20. *Make other people laugh*
21. *Paint and awaken your artsy side*

Those are enough to get you started! The time is now! You must shake yourself loose from your rut. Wake up and stop being so moody. Life is too short for you to live so depressed, angry and bored! Make it a goal to never again lose your playfulness. You will be so healthy if you can learn to start laughing and having fun with your life. Do things out of the ordinary! Stop allowing yourself to remain stuck and bored. Go for a run! Start juicing daily! Get good rest! Wake up happy! Play upbeat music! Connect with God! Smile at others! Laugh at yourself. Laugh with your family. Tell funny stories and laugh. Make your home the happiest and most exciting place on earth. Make memories and give your children the gift of being a joyful and fun parent! Even if you are a grandparent, don't be the moody one! Be the one that is fun to be around. Don't be the grandparent who is negative and cold. Your grandkids will idolize you and want to stay at your house if you are fun and funny. There is so much life for us to live. It's going to happen so fast as it is. We might as well start having fun and enjoying ourselves more!

5. Surround yourself with Healthy People

Of course there are actually many things that we must do in order to live a healthy lifestyle. However, these five are absolutely necessary if you plan on living a healthy life. I've coached so many people to lose weight and those that really did it right and maintained a healthy lifestyle were those that had a strong support group. It really does matter who you associate with and spend time with. If you want to be healthy, you need to spend time with healthy people. That is why it's so good for you to have a gym membership. While you may not feel confident in your own body to go to the gym, go anyway. You may not have the best body in the gym, but if you go with enthusiasm, then you'll even gain the respect of others who are working out in the gym, even if they do have a better body than you. You'll meet other likeminded, healthy people at the gym. It's also good to shop at healthy places such as whole foods and health food stores. Again, you'll be in the right environment and meet the type of people that you want to surround yourself with. Another good place to meet healthy people is at juice bars and health food stores. Granted you may not become best friends with everyone that you meet at these types of places, but you will feel a kinship with other people who are on the same journey that you are. I'm going to share two very powerful scriptures from the Bible that help support this principle:

"Can two walk together, except they be agreed?"- Amos 3:3

"He that walketh with wise men shall be wise: but a companion of fools shall be destroyed." - Proverbs 13:20

The first scripture in Amos tells us, "Can two walk together, except they be agreed?" It's much easier to walk closely with people in life that you have more in common with. This is why it's so important to associate closely with other people that place a high value on their health and take care of their body by juicing and exercising on a consistent basis. The next scripture in Proverbs is one of my personal favorites and one that I teach my son Caleb on a regular basis. God said, "He that walks with wise men shall be wise!" What is the principle here? The principle is that you literally will become what you walk closely with. For example, if you walk with positive people, you'll become positive! If you walk with healthy people, you'll be healthy. What happens if you walk with negative people? That is right, you'll be negative! Make sure that you ask your family to join with you on this health journey. I really hope that you are reading this book with your spouse! I hope you call a family meeting and declare that your home is going to be a healthy home! I hope that you do this together! If you want to lose weight, find a buddy with the same goal and help each other by encouraging each other and holding each other accountable.

Whatever you do, don't be the one to discourage those who want to be healthy. If your spouse wants to lose weight and live a healthy lifestyle, be their biggest encourager and support. If your best friend wants to eat healthy, don't suggest that you guys meet at McDonalds for lunch. Don't tempt those who are trying to do better. Be respectful and supportive of their health and weight loss journey!

Chapter 4

Foods that Fight Cancer

One of the things that I'm very passionate about is living an Alkaline lifestyle, and I am very focused on making sure that I eat the things that keep my body Alkaline. "The Alkaline Diet Recipe Book" says that after digestion, food leaves a residue in the body. The pH of this residue varies depending on the type of food eaten, and can be acidic, neutral or alkaline. The residue affects the pH of the blood, and acidic blood can lead to conditions such as high blood pressure, stroke, cancer and heart disease. Eating more alkaline foods cause the pH of the blood to stabilize at a slightly alkaline pH between 7.35 and 7.45.

The body has a pH balance that determines the amount of acid and alkalinity present in your system. Being highly acidic may not necessarily be life threatening, but it can cause various symptoms. Examples of these include low energy levels, fatigue, irritability, headaches, recurring infections and dry skin. Eating foods that are high in acid can exacerbate these symptoms; therefore, knowing what to avoid can be helpful. It's been said that it's extremely rare and almost impossible to get cancer when you keep your body alkaline. Here is a list of high alkaline foods:

1. *Okra*
2. *Water with lemon*
3. *Parsley*
4. *Spinach*
5. *Broccoli*
6. *Celery*
7. *Garlic*
8. *Barley Grass*
9. *Green Beans*
10. *Lima Beans*

11. Carrots
12. Beets
13. Lettuce
14. Zucchini
15. Dried figs and raisins
16. Dates
17. Grapes
18. Papaya
19. Kiwi
20. Hazelnuts and almonds
21. Green Tea
22. Tomatoes
23. Avocados
24. Limes
25. Grapefruits
26. Soy Beans

The good news is that most of this can be juiced. I'm very intentional on making sure that at least 80% of my eating and juicing is comprised of foods that are high in alkaline. Here is a list of foods that are highly acidic and should be avoided or eaten in moderation:

1. Eggs (organic, cage free is acceptable)
2. Certain gourmet cheeses (goat and feta are good)
3. Yogurt (in moderation)
4. Dairy milk (almond and rice milk are better for you)
5. Sour cream
6. Proteins – mainly red meat
7. Junk food
8. Artificial sweeteners (avoid all of these)
9. Ice Cream
10. Soda
11. High Fructose Corn Syrup
12. Corn
13. Olives

14. *Canned fruits*
15. *Glazed fruits*
16. *White bread*
17. *White rice*
18. *White pasta*
19. *Biscuits*
20. *Bagels*
21. *Donuts*
22. *Pastries*
23. *Crackers*
24. *Cream cheese*
25. *Cottage cheese*
26. *Butter*
27. *Bacon*
28. *Sausage*
29. *Ham*
30. *Corned Beef*

Again, you can eat these foods in moderation, but they definitely do not need to be a part of your daily routine of eating. Please take me serious on this. I'm asking you to consider making a commitment to living a lifestyle that is high in alkaline. You'll feel better and will be a lot healthier if you avoid these highly acidic foods.

I also want you to consider the following list of foods that are strong in fighting cancer. I've studied my brains out about this and have come up with a list of foods that are healthy for you and that will help fight against cancer. Please take this serious! I know this will help you live a healthier life.

Matt's Top 35 Cancer-Fighting Foods

1. *Turmeric*
2. *Blueberries*
3. *Strawberries*

4. Green Tea
5. Tomatoes
6. Grapes
7. Grapefruit
8. Garlic
9. Cabbage
10. Broccoli
11. Brussels sprouts
12. Collard greens
13. Oolong Tea
14. White Tea
15. Omega 3's
16. Salmon
17. Lemons
18. Grapefruit
19. Dark Chocolate
20. Carrots
21. Spinach
22. Fresh ground flax seed
23. Blackberries
24. Onions
25. Apples (Always remove the seeds.)
26. Artichoke
27. Avocado
28. Celery
29. Lentils
30. Alfalfa sprouts
31. Dark green leafy vegetables
32. Ginger
33. Whole grains
34. Pinto and red kidney beans
35. Cauliflower

I hate cancer! I hate what it does to people! I realize that it's one of the leading causes of deaths in America. I know we don't have all the answers and there are rare occasions when the mightiest are struck with this deadly disease and lose the battle. However, I'm calling for a war against cancer before it has a chance to grow in our body. Please fight it now! Fight it before you have it. Go on the offense and don't wait until the "wake up call" to get serious about your health. I want you to become a health nut. Yes! I said it, "HEALTH NUT!" You should be absolutely crazy about your health. You only get one body and one life! Don't neglect your health. You'll lay in that hospital bed with so much regret if you don't listen to the whispers. Someone one said, "You'll have to listen to the screams if you ignore the whispers!" You are hearing a whisper right now as you read this book. It's God's way of giving you that little whisper and reminding you that your health is nothing to take lightly. Here is a list of the top cancer-causing foods based on my opinion and research:

1. *All charred food*
2. *Well-done red meat. Little or no red meat is healthiest choice*
3. *Sugar*
4. *Heavily salted, smoked and pickled foods*
5. *Sodas/soft drinks*
6. *French fries, chips and snack foods that contain trans fats*
7. *Food and drink additives such as aspartame*
8. *Excess alcohol*
9. *Farmed fish, which contains higher levels of toxins such as PCBs.*
10. *Microwave popcorn*
11. *Non-organic fruits*
12. *Canned tomatoes*
13. *Processed meats*
14. *Hydrogenated oils*
15. *Highly processed white flours*
16. *GMO's*

I would avoid foods and drinks on this list at all cost. It's just not worth the risk. There have been many studies that prove that these types of foods and drinks will put you at high risk and more vulnerable to cancer. Isn't it amazing that there are little choices that we could be making on a daily basis that will determine our health? I'm so intentional on doing my part in helping the world become a healthier place. I don't believe we should live our lives in fear or panic that if we have a piece of cake that we'll end up with cancer. However, I do believe that we should live our life in extreme caution when it comes to what we put in our bodies. That is why juicing is so safe and healthy. We can assure that we are giving our bodies the nutrients that it needs to stay alive and disease free.

Chapter 5

My Best Advice for Overweight and Unhealthy People

I work with about 10-15 people a week as a Weight Loss Coach. It's by far one of my favorite things in the world to do. I LOVE helping people lose weight and get healthy. However, I do want to point out the title of this chapter, "My Best Advice for Overweight and Unhealthy People!" I've actually worked with a lot of people that were "skinny" but very unhealthy in their lifestyle. I tell my clients all the time, "My goal is not just to get you to lose weight, but my goal is to help you get healthy. If you focus on getting healthy, then you'll lose the weight and be able to keep it off." I see people go on diets all the time and lose a significant amount of weight, yet sadly, because they never have dealt with their emotional issues or changed their lifestyle, they end up gaining back the weight that was lost plus more.

I'm sure by now you can see that I believe in making lists. It's one of the easiest ways to clear your mind and get more control in your life. The simple act of making a list will help you stay on target with your goals and produce greater results in your life. I'm going to give you a list of things to do in order to live a healthy lifestyle.

1. Eliminate Stress –

This is more important than any supplement and vitamin that you could take. In fact, neglect to do this and you cannot take enough supplements or juice to heal the damage that will be done to your immune system. This number one secret to building a healthy immune system is more important than anything you could possibly do. It's important that you start doing things that will help you eliminate stress, such as: (1) Physical exercise, (2) Meditation, (3) Not allowing yourself to worry about the future, (4) Getting regular massages – at least twice a month, and (5) Physical rest. Take more vacations, days off and rest your mind and body from the stress of life. For me personally, nothing reduces stress more than prayer and spending time in the presence of God.

Develop a Schedule for Eating and Juicing

Rarely have I ever seen somebody get healthy or live a healthy life without having a routine or schedule of some sort. When you get into the habit of juicing or eating every 2-3 hours, you'll notice that you will start to do it without even thinking about it.

Doing this will also help you stop binge eating or eating more than you should. There is something about knowing you'll be eating again in 2-3 hours that keeps you from feeling deprived. There is a mental battle that we all face when it comes to eating healthy. Many feel that they are doomed and will never be able to enjoy "normal" food again. Friends, I'm actually the coach that will help you eat healthy in such a way that you'll want to eat healthy and will enjoy this new healthy lifestyle.

You need to start eating about 4-6 times a day. Don't ever skip breakfast except when you are fasting. Make smaller and healthier choices throughout your day such as berries, fruits, carrots, a turkey wrap, salad, juice, a bowl of soup, plate of broccoli, some nuts, grapes, chicken, fish or other white meat. Be very careful about the amount of red meat you put into your body because over the long term, it will damage your immune system. Here is a good sample daily schedule that I follow:

Daily Schedule for Healthy Eating:

6:00 am – Eat a bowl of Oatmeal and Eggs
9:00 am – Drink a Protein Shake or make a Juice or Smoothie

12:00 noon – Eat a Salad or Turkey wrap for lunch
3:00 pm – Drink a juice from my recipe book
6:00 pm – Eat Organic Chicken or Fish with grilled vegetables
9:00 pm – Eat some Nuts or a Green juice

If you'll notice a trend, I usually eat or drink a juice every 3 hours. I always feel full, and maintaining this schedule gives me more energy without feeling sluggish. The best advice that I can give you is to develop a routine and get into the habit of eating smaller portions every 2-3 hours. If you are overweight and desire to lose weight the healthy way, don't ever starve yourself. I know some who think that they will lose weight if they just eat one big meal a day. It's simply not true, nor is it healthy for your body to eat this way.

I do recommend that you eat breakfast every morning and don't skip it. Many people get in the bad habit of skipping meals, but breakfast is the worst one to skip. I coach my clients to get into the habit of eating oatmeal every morning. Oatmeal is a whole grain, and eating whole grains can lower your risk for several diseases, including high blood pressure and type 2 diabetes. Avoid prepackaged oatmeal that may be high in both sodium and sugar and lower in beneficial fiber. You are looking for "whole grain oats" when buying your oatmeal. I am always a fan of buying organic anything. Eating oatmeal can lower cholesterol. Mayoclinic.com even recommends oatmeal as one of the top five foods to eat to improve your cholesterol numbers. Oatmeal is a good source of fiber. Oatmeal contains a wide variety of vitamins, minerals and antioxidants and is a good source of protein, complex carbohydrates and iron.

Matt's Top 10 Oatmeal Recipes:

Oatmeal, Almond Milk, Cinnamon, Bananas

Oatmeal, Almond Milk, Coconut Oil, Almonds

Oatmeal, Almond Milk, Strawberries, Bananas

Oatmeal, Almond Milk, Granola, Blueberries

Oatmeal, Almond Milk, Raspberries, Bananas

Oatmeal, Almond Milk, Peanut Butter, Organic Jelly

Oatmeal, Almond Milk, Sliced Peaches

Oatmeal, Almond Milk, Cinnamon, Raisins, Granola

Oatmeal, Almond Milk, Sunflower Seeds, Almonds, Pecans, Blueberries

Oatmeal, Almond Milk, Pumpkin Spice, Bananas

Remember, you don't want to add sugar. There are some occasions that I'll be craving a good old-fashioned peanut butter and jelly sandwich, because I don't eat much bread, although I flat LOVE it. Instead, I make a bowl of oatmeal and put a scoop of peanut butter and jelly in it, and I feel so much better than if I eat all that bread. It gives me my PB&J fix, and I'm happy.

2. Get into the Habit of Daily Exercise

I always start all of my clients off with a 30-minute walk everyday. The secret is to do it daily and really work hard to do it at the same exact time everyday. You'd be surprised how much better you'll start feeling when you do this on a daily basis. One of the things that will help you with this is to never cheat, make excuses or allow yourself to skip your daily exercise.

It is a proven fact that people who keep their body moving and get good physical exercise are less prone to get sick and tend to live happier, healthier and longer lives. Friends, we get 24 hours in a day. You have plenty of time to give at least 30 minutes to an hour to good physical exercise. One of the best ways to stay consistent with your exercise is to have an exercise buddy or perhaps your spouse or kids to work out with you everyday.

3. Drink Tea Daily

Drinking Tea is one of the healthiest habits that you can add to your lifestyle. Those who drink the right kinds of tea will see major results in their health. Health experts have long vouched for the long-ranging health benefits of drinking tea. Not only does Tea help detoxify the body, but it also keeps the skin hydrated, helps with weight management, is good for the hair and will give you increased energy throughout the day. Here are the top benefits of drinking Tea:

1. *Tea contains antioxidants.*
2. *Tea has less caffeine than coffee.*
3. *Tea is good for your bones.*
4. *Tea bolsters your immune system.*
5. *Tea protects against cancer.*
6. *Tea helps keep you hydrated.*
7. *Tea may reduce your risk of heart attack and stroke.*
8. *Tea increases your metabolism.*
9. *Tea can boost exercise endurance.*
10. *Tea is linked with a lower risk of Parkinson's disease.*
11. *Tea can be beneficial to those with Type 2 diabetes.*
12. *Tea helps with weight loss.*
13. *Tea helps reduce stress and anxiety.*
14. *Tea helps with bad breath.*
15. *Tea helps reduce inflammation.*
16. *Tea will help detoxify the body.*

17. Tea will keep the skin looking healthy.
18. Tea can prevent tooth decay.

As you can see, those reasons alone are worthy enough for you to stop turning to Diet Coke and coffee. If you start drinking Tea on a daily basis, you'll reap all of the benefits listed above. It's amazing what Tea can do for the body! Drinking tea is fun, relaxing and energizing! You'll actually even start to enjoy the process of making it. Following is a list of my recommendations of the healthiest teas to drink:

1. Silver Needle Tea
2. Oolong Tea
3. Gyokuro Green Tea
4. Matcha Green Tea
5. Black Tea
6. Peppermint Tea
7. Ginger Tea
8. Chamomile Tea (Drink before bed)
9. Rooibos Tea
10. Milk Thistle and Dandelion Tea

Matt's Best Advice for New Tea Drinkers:

1. Avoid Lipton tea or bottles or cans of store-bought tea

2. Avoid drinking tea from tea bags if at all possible

3. Drink loose leaf tea and store it in tin cans – it keeps nutritional value when stored in cans or jars

4. Don't over-steep your tea and burn it. Here is a chart to follow:

Green Tea – 2 minutes
White Tea – 4 minutes

43

Oolong Tea – 3 minutes
Black Tea – 3 minutes
Rooibos Tea– 5 minutes
Herbal Tea – 5 minutes

5. Don't EVER add sugar to your tea. Stop drinking sweet tea.

6. If you need to add sweetener – use stevia or agave (in moderation.)

7. Pour your tea over Ice as often as you desire. I drink a lot of my tea over ice.

8. Don't forget that loose leaf tea can be infused many times

    White and Green Tea – infuse about 4 times
    Black Tea – infuse about 5 times
    Oolong Tea – infuse about 5 times
    Rooibos Tea – infuse about 3 times
    Herbal Tea – infuse about 3 times

9. Mix Silver Needle with flavored Rooibos Teas. One of my favorites is Silver Needle and Blueberry Rooibos. It's so refreshing!

10. Have fun with your tea experience and visit as many teashops as you can. Keep learning about tea and enjoy the journey. Tea is a gift from God.

4. Become Emotionally Healthy

I strongly advise for you to really do the work of becoming emotionally healthy. This is easier said than done. However, if you are willing to do whatever it takes to become emotionally whole, then you will have an easier time with weight loss. I've worked with a lot of people who were overweight and unhealthy. Most of them struggle with extreme low self-esteem and emotional baggage.

The secret to emotional healing starts with you finally loving yourself. While an entire book could be written about this subject alone, I do want to give you a few principles that will help you to heal emotionally. The reason why it's so important to heal and become emotionally strong is because most people that gain weight also struggle with emotionally eating. Almost all of my previous clients had a major battle with binge eating because they didn't know how to cope with the negative emotions. How to heal emotionally:

1. *Forgive and let go of all bitterness.*
2. *Love yourself.*
3. *Let go of anger and resentment.*
4. *Stop being a victim.*
5. *Think positive and happy thoughts.*
6. *Laugh more and develop a good sense of humor.*
7. *Let go of stress and anxiety.*

5. Speak Affirmations Daily

Speaking your affirmations could be the deciding factor of whether you have a health breakthrough or not. Affirmations provide a massive boost to health, energy and vitality. If you combine these positive affirmations with taking care of yourself, eating right, juicing and exercise, you will transform yourself into a healthy person.

The Bible says, "Life and Death are in the power of the tongue!" Speaking these affirmations will help you overcome deeply held negative beliefs and thought patterns. You words are that powerful. Don't try to change your lifestyle without speaking affirmations on a daily basis. I usually speak mine right before bed, first thing in the morning and while I'm working out. By speaking them three times each day, you will begin to feel a conquering power over bad habits and an unhealthy lifestyle. Affirmations will help you stick to your healthy lifestyle, say no to temptation, and eat nourishing foods.

It's important to use "I am" statements so that you can demonstrate a certainty and confidence that is lacking when you choose to use expressions like "I want to be" or "I can be!" Think about it for a moment. Wanting to be something, have something or believing that you deserve something doesn't ensure that you'll get it. The only thing that can guarantee you results is a personal conviction that you are already devoted to taking action. That is the power that comes from saying "I AM!" It signals to your subconscious mind that there is no doubt about whether or not something is possible. It underlines the belief that what you want is already a work in progress.

Affirmations are positive statements stated in the present. Speaking your affirmations in the present helps your brain overwrite negative thoughts that may be holding you back. Present-focused affirmations help you "live" the emotional feelings that go along with being healthy, energetic, positive, optimistic, diligent and enthusiastic! Affirmations will only work if you are serious about using them on a regular basis, which is why I say my affirmations three times a day. Here are my 21 Affirmations that I personally speak on a daily basis:

1. *I am firmly committed to staying active and healthy.*
2. *I am attracting health into my life.*
3. *I have a strong and healthy body.*
4. *I enjoy exercising daily.*
5. *I am grateful for my perfect health.*
6. *I am enjoying the process of juicing.*

7. I am able to say no to sugar and bad foods.
8. I am highly focused on living a healthy lifestyle.
9. I find it easy to eat right and make healthy choices.
10. I am happy with myself and love myself.
11. I am enjoying healthy salads.
12. I am happy about living a disease and sickness-free life.
13. I drink plenty of good, clean water everyday.
14. I am living a stress-free lifestyle.
15. I am grateful that I have a positive attitude.
16. I allow myself enough sleep to rest my body every night.
17. I am able to afford organic foods and a healthy lifestyle.
18. I live my life with radiant good health.
19. I rest peacefully, knowing that my body is healing.
20. I have abundant energy and a healthy immune system.
21. I am full of joy, happiness, life and have a peaceful mind.

I speak those affirmations three times a day! It's important to note that you should speak these out loud with enthusiasm and conviction. You have to feel it while you speak it and allow your heart to believe it deeply. You are doing more than just positive speaking.

Chapter 6

Benefits of Fruits and Vegetables

Eating/juicing vegetables provides health benefits – people who eat/juice more vegetables and fruits as part of an overall healthy lifestyle are likely to have a reduced risk of some chronic diseases. Vegetables provide nutrients vital for health and maintenance of your body.

A lifestyle of consuming vegetables and fruits may reduce the risk of heart disease, including heart attack and stroke! Eating a diet rich in some vegetables and fruits as an overall healthy diet may protect against certain types of cancers. A lifestyle of eating foods containing fiber, such as some vegetables and fruits, may reduce the risk of heart disease, obesity, and type 2 diabetes. Eating vegetables and fruits rich in potassium as an overall healthy diet may lower blood pressure, reduce the risk of developing kidney stones, and help to decrease bone loss.

Most vegetables are naturally low in fat and calories. None have cholesterol. Vegetables are important sources of many nutrients, including potassium, dietary fiber, vitamin A, and vitamin C. Dietary fiber from vegetables eaten as part of an overall healthy diet, helps reduce blood cholesterol levels. Fiber is important for proper bowel function. It helps reduce constipation and diverticulitis.

There are so many benefits of eating/juicing fruits and vegetables. I always wanted a list of all the benefits of the healthiest fruits and vegetables. I didn't want to read a whole book to find out the benefit of a vegetable. I wanted bullet points of the benefits. Therefore, I decided to put it in my book. Here are the health benefits of each one:

Health Benefits of Fruits

APPLES:

The fibers of an apple help to clean your teeth and palate of bacteria and food residue. Apples can help lower the chances of developing asthma and diabetes. They are rich in Vitamin A, B, C, K, alpha-hydroxy acid (malic acid), phytonutrients, flavonoids, and phenols; they are protective against cell and tissue damage, contain powerful antioxidant activity, and promote skin rejuvenation.

1. *Alzheimer prevention*
2. *Lung cancer prevention*
3. *Breast cancer prevention*
4. *Bone protection*
5. *Colon cancer prevention*
6. *Liver cancer prevention*
7. *Weight Loss*
8. *Prevent Stroke*
9. *Boost your immune system*
10. *Prevent gallstones*
11. *Detoxify your liver*
12. *Weight Loss*
13. *Asthma Prevention*
14. *Cure constipation*
15. *Relieve from Hemorrhoids*
16. *Help reduce wrinkles*
17. *Prevent Cataracts*

BLACKBERRIES:

They are considered a powerful antioxidant that may help to reduce risk of certain cancers. Blackberries are rich in vitamins, minerals and fiber. They are also low in calories, carbohydrates, and fat.

1. *Cancer prevention*
2. *Lower risk of heart disease*
3. *Skin health – Younger looking skin*
4. *Relieve bloating*
5. *Aid in maintaining bowel regularity*
6. *Good source of Vitamin K*
7. *Control Diabetes*
8. *Boost immune system*
9. *Relieve Post Menopausal Symptoms*

BLUEBERRIES:

Blueberries are loaded with many antioxidants, which help to lower the risk of developing Alzheimer's and Parkinson's disease. Blueberries are also rich in vitamin B2, C and E, manganese and fiber.

1. *Cancer prevention*
2. *Slow the progress of Hepatitis C*
3. *Reduce risk of heart disease*
4. *Prevent urinary tract infections*
5. *Lower cholesterol*
6. *Reduce inflammation*
7. *Eye health*
8. *Improve Memory*
9. *Reduce risk of Breast Cancer*
10. *Regulate Blood Sugar*
11. *Prevent Constipation*
12. *Improve Bone Health*
13. *Reduce Belly Fat*
14. *Slow down aging – Prevent premature wrinkles*

BANANAS:

Bananas are a rich source of potassium that can help to maintain a healthy blood pressure level and are a good source of vitamins and minerals, as well as fiber.

1. *Lower blood pressure*
2. *Bone health*
3. *High nutrient absorption*
4. *Healthy digestive tract*
5. *Cancer prevention*
6. *Vitamin B6 – Anti-inflammatory agent*
7. *Reduce Heart Disease*
8. *Prevent constipation*
9. *Help in Diarrhea Treatment*
10. *Decrease risk of Stroke*
11. *Provide instant energy*
12. *Prevent insomnia*
13. *Help overcome depression*
14. *Protect against Muscle Cramps*
15. *Stress relief*

GRAPES:

Resveratrol, an antioxidant found in grapes, may help to lower the risk of developing blood clots and also reduce high blood pressure. This antioxidant may also help prevent heart diseases. Resveratrol has also been seen to help arrest the spread of cancer cells, especially in breast, colon and stomach cancers. Grapes have a high content of vitamin A, B1, B2, B6 and C. They also contain many health-promoting flavonoids.

1. *Reduce risk of Heart Attack*
2. *Cancer prevention*
3. *Antibacterial and Antiviral Properties – infection protection*

4. *Anti-Aging*
5. *Lung health*
6. *Increased Energy*
7. *Eye Health – prevent loss of vision*
8. *Cure migraine*
9. *Cure constipation*
10. *Prevent Breast Cancer*
11. *Lower Blood Cholesterol*
12. *Boost immune system*
13. *Cure indigestion*
14. *Reduce skin wrinkles*

STRAWBERRIES:

Strawberries contain a chemical compound called phenols. Anthocyanin, a particular phenol abundantly found in strawberries, lends the rich red color to the fruit. Strawberries are rich in fiber, flavonoids, anti-oxidants, potassium and vitamins B2, B5 and B6.

1. *Lower blood pressure*
2. *Curb overeating*
3. *Strong in antioxidants*
4. *Anti-inflammatory*
5. *Cancer prevention*
6. *Healthy eyes*
7. *Vigorous Vitamin C*
8. *Bone Health*
9. *Reduce risk of type 2 diabetes*
10. *Boost immune system*
11. *Prevent constipation*
12. *Teeth whitening*
13. *Skin repairing*
14. *Improve complexion*

RASPBERRIES:

The delicious, soft, and juicy raspberry is among the most popular berries grown all over the world.

1. *Eye Health – improve vision*
2. *Boost immune system*
3. *Reduce risk of Cancer*
4. *Reduce risk of Heart Attack*
5. *Strong in Antioxidants*
6. *Anti-inflammatory properties*
7. *Reduce obesity*
8. *Prevent overeating*
9. *Low in Calories*
10. *Slow down the aging process*
11. *Help the skin glow*
12. *Reduce wrinkles*

WATERMELON:

Watermelon is one of the most delicious and nutrient-rich fruits. It's so good for juicing and is one of my favorites to use in my juicing recipes. The water content in watermelon is extremely high at 92%. It is rich in beta-carotene, folate, vitamin C, and vitamin B5.

1. *Lowers Bad Cholesterol*
2. *Prevents Cancer*
3. *Kidney Health – Detoxifies toxins from the kidney*
4. *Bone Health*
5. *Boosts Immune System*
6. *Treats Erectile Dysfunction*
7. *Improves Male Fertility*
8. *Helps in Weight Loss*
9. *Increases Brain Power*
10. *Slows down aging process*

11. *Good source of Vitamin C and Vitamin A*
12. *Eye Health*
13. *Reduces muscle pain*
14. *Reduces Risk of Heart Attack*
15. *Low in Calories*
16. *Helps with Bladder Problems*

PINEAPPLE:

Pineapple is a sweet, sharp and juicy source of Vitamin C and is also a great aid to digestion. Eating/juicing pineapple is good for your body both inside and out – eating a few slices of pineapple a day can defend your body from harmful free radicals and disease, and help your digestion by cleaning the body's organs and blood.

1. *Improves Digestion*
2. *Prevents coughs and colds*
3. *Prevents Blood Clots*
4. *Reduces risk of Heart Disease*
5. *Lowers Blood Cholesterol*
6. *Relieves Nausea*
7. *Kills Tumor Cells*
8. *Cures Constipation*
9. *Fights against Intestinal Worms*
10. *Slows down Aging*
11. *Prevents Migraine Headaches*
12. *Strengthens the Immune System*
13. *Eye Health – Prevents Age Related Macular Degeneration*

PEACHES:

Peaches are juicy, sweet, and nutritious. But more than that, peaches are good for your body's overall health and can act as a home remedy for many ailments.

1. *Help lose weight*
2. *Healthy looking skin*
3. *Lower Cholesterol*
4. *Reduce High Blood Pressure*
5. *Slow progression of eye diseases*
6. *Prevent Cancer*
7. *Vitamin K*
8. *Reduce Risk of Heart Disease*
9. *Prevent Constipation*
10. *Prevent Kidney Stones*

GRAPEFRUIT:

Grapefruit doesn't only contain vitamin C, which is commonly known to be protective against cold or flu. This juicy fruit also contains citrus acid, natural sugars, and essential oils. It has high amounts of vitamin C, and smaller amounts of vitamin A, B complex, E and K.

1. *Reduces Risk of Breast Cancer*
2. *Boosts Immune System*
3. *Prevents Colds and Flu*
4. *Reduces Risk of Diabetes*
5. *Prevents Constipation*
6. *Increases Energy and Reduces Fatigue*
7. *Reduces Fever*
8. *Helps Relive Sore Throats and Soothes Coughs*
9. *Prevents Cancer*
10. *Helps with Weight Loss*
11. *Reduces Cholesterol Problems*
12. *Prevents Kidney Stones*
13. *Healthy Heart – Prevents Heart Disease*
14. *Prevents Infections*
15. *Prevents Respiratory Problems and Asthma*
16. *Liver Cleanser*

17. *Improves Eyesight*
18. *Prevents Skin Dryness and Wrinkles*
19. *Soft and Glowing Skin*
20. *Reduces Gum Problems*

KIWI:

The main nutritional benefit of kiwifruit is its exceptional vitamin C content, which is even higher than that of oranges and lemons. In addition to vitamin C, kiwifruit is packed with many other healthy nutrients, including vitamin A and E, potassium, copper, iron and magnesium. It also contains a relatively high amount of fiber as well.

1. *Strong in Antioxidants*
2. *Good for bone, tooth and gum health*
3. *Prevents Constipation*
4. *Protects sperms from genetic damage that may cause birth defects*
5. *Helps Reduce Blood Cholesterol*
6. *Prevents Heart Disease*
7. *Boosts Immune System*
8. *Prevents Muscle Cramps and Improves Muscle Strength*
9. *Increases Concentration and Relieves Mental Fatigue*
10. *Reduces the Risk of Stomach Cancer*

ORGANGES:

The orange is one of the most common and popular fruits. It is well liked because of its easy availability all year round; it has dense nutrition, and it tastes so good. The best oranges for juicing (sweeter ones) include Valencia, Navel and Jaffa. Oranges are an excellent source of vitamin C and flavonoids. In addition, oranges are a good source of vitamin A, the B vitamins, amino acids, calcium, zinc, manganese, iron and potassium.

1. *Prevent Cancer*
2. *Reduce Cholesterol*
3. *Prevent Constipation*
4. *Reduce Risk of Heart Disease*
5. *Boost The Immune System*
6. *Prevent Kidney Stones*
7. *Healthy Skin – Natural Glow to Your Skin*
8. *Reduce Risk of Stomach Cancer*
9. *Protection against Viral Infections*
10. *Reduce Risk of Arthritis*
11. *Maintain Bone and Teeth Health*
12. *Cure Acne and Pimples*
13. *Prevent Premature Aging*

LEMONS AND LIMES:

The nutritional benefits of limes do not differ much from those of lemons. They are both excellent sources of vitamin C, BC, flavonoids, potassium, and limonene.

1. *Reduce Fever*
2. *Balance pH*
3. *Good source of Alkaline*
4. *Prevent Cancer*
5. *Aid in Digestion*
6. *Soothe Sore Throats*
7. *Prevent Kidney Stones*
8. *Help with Weight Loss*
9. *Improve Immunity*
10. *Help Improve Liver Function and Flush Toxins*
11. *Reduce High Blood Pressure*
12. *Aid in Relieving Respiratory and Breathing Disorders*
13. *Improve Indigestion*
14. *Refresh Breath and Dental Care*
15. *Healthy Glowing Skin*

16. Help with Weight Loss
17. Dissolve Kidney and Gall Stones
18. Increase Energy
19. Boost The Immune System

PEARS:

Pears are an excellent source of water-soluble fiber. They contain vitamin A, C, E and B1 and B2. Pears are also rich in copper, potassium and phosphorus.

1. Prevent High Blood Pressure and Stroke
2. Prevent Cancer
3. Help Lower Cholesterol Levels
4. Promote Healthy Colon
5. Prevent Constipation
6. Increase Energy
7. Reduce Fever
8. Boost Immune System
9. Reduce Inflammation
10. Help with Shortness of Breath
11. Nourish the Throat and Prevent Throat Problems
12. Improve Digestion
13. Help to prevent Birth Defects during Pregnancy
14. Healthy and Glowing Skin

The Health Benefits of Vegetables

BROCOLI:

Broccoli is low in calories and especially rich in vitamins A, C, K, B6 and E, calcium, potassium and magnesium. Broccoli is strong in antioxidants and is an excellent food for cancer prevention, particularly breast, prostrate, colon, lung and cervical cancer.

1. *Prevents possible birth defects*
2. *Promotes Good Colon Health*
3. *Protects from Eye Disorders*
4. *Boosts the Immune System*
5. *Helps boost liver and skin's detoxification abilities*
6. *Helps Stomach Disorders*
7. *Helps reduce the size of Tumors*
8. *Bone building*
9. *Powerful Antioxidant*
10. *Helps with Weight Loss – Low Calorie*
11. *Reduces Allergy Reaction and Inflammation*
12. *Anti-Ageing Benefits*
13. *Helps Regulate Blood Pressure and Reduces Bad Cholesterol*
14. *Helps Prevent Heart Attacks*
15. *Great source of Fiber*

KALE:

Kale has been crowned as the "queen of greens," and could be referred to as the queen of Vitamin A. Kale has over 100% of the average person's daily Vitamin A and C requirement. I would crawl on my hands and knees across America if I could convince people to start juicing and eating Kale.

1. *High Fiber Content*
2. *Great source of Calcium*
3. *Good for Bone Health*
4. *Brain Health*
5. *Prevents Cancer*
6. *Reduces Cholesterol*
7. *Detoxifying*
8. *Highly Alkaline*
9. *Reduces Inflammation*
10. *High in Protein*
11. *Promotes Healthy Skin*

12. *Healthy Eyes and Vision*
13. *Helps with Weight Loss*
14. *Iron Content*
15. *Strong in Vitamin C*
16. *Helps in Prevention of Lung and Oral Cavity Disease*
17. *Packed with Omega 3 and Omega 6 Fatty Acids*

TOMATO:

Tomatoes provide almost 20 percent of the vitamin intake necessary per serving. It is rich in potassium, vitamin A, flavonoid B complex, thiamine, folate and iron.

1. *Prevents Cancer*
2. *Strong Antioxidant*
3. *Helps the Body Detox*
4. *Healthy for Bones*
5. *Enhances the Digestive Function*
6. *Improves Heart Health*
7. *Relives Stress, Tiredness and Fatigue*
8. *Healthy Skin*
9. *Helps Regulate Blood Sugar*
10. *Improves Your Vision and Prevents Blindness*
11. *Makes your Hair Look Better*
12. *Prevents Kidney Stones and Gallstones*
13. *Helps Reduce Chronic Pain*
14. *Anti-Inflammatory*
15. *Helps Lose Weight*
16. *Good for Cell Repair and Muscle Building*
17. *Less Fat Content*

BEETS:

Beets are not my favorite vegetable to juice. However, I discipline myself to juice beets on weekly basis because they are so healthy for you. Beets are high in folic acid and manganese. Beets are an insane source of vitamins and minerals.

1. *Lower Blood Pressure*
2. *Boost your Stamina - Improve Physical Activity*
3. *Anti-Cancer Properties*
4. *Reduce Inflammation*
5. *Rich in Valuable Nutrients and Fiber*
6. *Help Purify your Blood and your Liver*
7. *Help your Mental Health and Can Cure Depression*
8. *High Source of Energy*
9. *Strong in Antioxidants*
10. *Reduce risk for Arthritis and Kidney Stones*
11. *Very Healthy for Pregnant Ladies – Prevent Birth Defects*
12. *Boost the Immune System*

GARLIC:

Garlic is well known as a natural health remedy that has long been used to treat various ailments. It is recommended that adults consume no more than one clove two-three times a day and that children have one quarter to one half a clove, once or twice a day. Garlic is packed with vitamins and nutrients. Some of these include vitamins A, B, B2 and C, as well as protein, potassium, calcium, zinc, iron and manganese.

1. *Cancer Prevention – Especially stomach and colon cancer*
2. *Prevents and Cures Colds*
3. *Decreases the risk of Heart Disease*
4. *Helps Lower Blood Sugar Level*
5. *Treats Fungal Infections – Athlete's Foot*
6. *Detoxifies the Blood*
7. *Strengthens the Immune System*
8. *Helps control Bacteria, Viral and Worm Infections*

9. *Prevents Blood Clots*
10. *Combats Allergies*
11. *Helps Reduce Toothaches*
12. *Helps with Weight Loss*

CARROTS:

Carrots are one of my favorite juice ingredients. In fact, Carrot and Apple juices are among my top favorite juices to combine. This combination has so many health benefits and is highly cleansing. Besides their delicious flavor, carrots contain high amounts of beta-carotene and other health-benefiting nutrients such as Vitamin A, minerals and antioxidants. Carrots offer several health benefits for the eyes, skin, digestive system and teeth.

1. *Reduce the Risk of Cancer*
2. *Relieve Constipation*
3. *Improve Eyesight*
4. *Anti-Inflammatory*
5. *Boost the Immune System*
6. *Helpful for Cleansing and Filtering the Kidneys*
7. *Enhance the quality of a nursing mother's breast milk*
8. *Nourish the Skin*
9. *Detox the Liver and Reduce Acne*
10. *Reduce the Risk of Heart Disease and Stroke*
11. *Dental Health – Prevent Tooth Decay*
12. *Prevent Ageing*
13. *Good Source of Calcium*
14. *Stimulate Hair Growth*
15. *Good Source of Fiber*

SPINACH:

I usually go through an entire container of Spinach about every two-three days. It's one of my favorite greens to juice and is usually included in most of my daily recipes.

1. *Cures Acne and Maintains Healthy Skin*
2. *Improves Complexion*
3. *Rich in Vitamin K – Maintains Healthy Bones*
4. *Lowers Hypertension – Helps Reduce Stress and Anxiety*
5. *Relaxes the Body*
6. *Corrects Behavioral and Cognitive Issues*
7. *Brain Health*
8. *Lowers Blood Pressure*
9. *Anti-inflammatory Properties*
10. *Boosts the Immune System*
11. *Beneficial for Weight Loss*
12. *Prevents Cancer*
13. *Promotes Eye Health*
14. *Prevents Heart Attacks*
15. *Protects against Ulcers*

I'm going to stop here. There are many other fruits and vegetables besides the ones that I've listed in this book. However, these are the predominant fruits and vegetables that I use for juicing. Therefore, I thought it necessary to share with you the benefits of each of these fruits and vegetables. Hopefully, the information presented in this chapter has awakened a fresh passion for you to pull out that juicer on a daily basis. As you can see, most all sickness and disease can be reduced if we would commit to juicing these fruits and vegetables on a daily basis. You would be a different person a year from today if you decided to juice at least twice a day. You would see such a difference in your body, skin and health.

Don't be stubborn anymore. Your life is too valuable to allow stubbornness to keep you from becoming a daily juicer. I know too many people who refuse to change just because they are too stubborn to listen. Don't wait until it's too late. Don't wait until you are lying in that Hospital bed with pain, illness and possibly death knocking at your door. The time is now. You have the answers in your hands right now. I've written this book for you. I want to help you get better and live a higher quality of life. Please read this chapter often and even try to memorize the benefits from each fruit and vegetable. Take it serious and get your health back.

Chapter 7

My Favorite Juicing Recipes

Let me start off by saying that I'm a huge fan of the Nutri-Bullet and Jack LaLane. There are so many juicers out there, and most of them will work and do what needs to be done for you to enjoy the benefits of fruits and vegetables. However, all of the recipes I have given in this book are for the Nutri-Bullet and the Jack LaLane. These are the two juicers that I use on a daily basis. I will give you recipes for both of them, but I will leave out the amount of fruits and vegetables that you should put in because you are going to have to be the judge of that as you learn what you like and what you don't. Juicing can be FUN, so make it an Adventure! Many people think getting healthy is a drudgery, but you are literally transforming your whole life. You will look better and feel better than you've ever felt. When you go to Whole Foods or wherever you shop, look upon it as a time of exploring new avenues to reclaiming your health.

The Jack LaLane is a great juicer to use for fruits and vegetables that are juicier. You'll get an instruction manual when you buy the Jack LaLane juicer. I recommend that you follow it. You will also see some recipes in there as well. Here is a list of fruits and vegetables that could go in the Jack LaLane. (Remember that you can get creative and make your own type of juices.)

1. *Carrots*
2. *Apples*
3. *Oranges*
4. *Lemons*
5. *Limes*
6. *Celery*
7. *Cucumber*

8. *Grapefruit*
9. *Pineapple*
10. *Ginger*
11. *Tomatoes*
12. *Watermelon*
13. *Pears*
14. *Beets*
15. *Cabbage*

All of these fruits and vegetables can be used in the Nutri-Bullet as well, but I like to use some of them in the Jack LaLane. Obviously the Jack LaLane takes a little longer to clean, but the quality of juice that you get from it is well worth the extra work.

Recipes for the Jack LaLane

Remember that you can put the amount that you think is necessary. I was going to tell you an amount of each, but I want you to have fun with it and mix it up according to what you like. I usually put a bowl under the spout and juice until the bowl is full. I usually have enough for 2-3 full glasses of juice when the bowl is full.

1. The Make-Grandma-Proud Juice

Carrots
Apples

2. Matt's Detox Juice

Oranges
Apples
Carrots
Celery
Ginger Root

3. Matt's Take-My-Breath-Away Juice

Apples
Watermelon
Limes
Lemon

4. Matt's Weight Loss Juice

Grapefruit
Watermelon
Lemons

5. Matt's Immune Booster Juice

Oranges
Lemons
Ginger

6. Matt's Green Monster Juice

Celery
Green Apples
Cucumber
Lime
Pear

7. Matt's Afternoon Pick-Me-Up Juice

Apples
Watermelon
Pineapple
Lemon

8. Matt's Make-Me-Feel-So-Clean drink

Watermelon
Limes

9. The Carrot Refresher Juice

Carrots
Apples
Ginger

10. The Caribbean Carrot Juice

Carrots
Pineapple
Grapefruit

11. The Carrot Blood Detox Juice

Carrots
Ginger
Celery
Apple

12. the Healthy Skin Juice

Pineapple
Cucumber
Apple

13. The Headache Relief Juice

Carrots
Apples
Beet
Grapefruit

14. Doctor Feel-Good Juice

Celery
Cucumber
Apple
Lemon
Ginger

Matt's Top Recipes for the Nutri-Bullet

I'm going to give you a lot of recipes for the Nutri-Bullet. However, you are always more than welcome to mix them up and try different combinations. It's supposed to be fun and something that you enjoy doing. Remember that when using the Nutri-Bullet, you put a little bit of each fruit or vegetable to the line and then fill it with water. I personally enjoy using coconut water.

1. The Green Refresh Juice

Spinach
Watermelon

2. Super Green Juice

Kale
Broccoli
Cucumber
Celery

Green Apple (if you need something sweet in it)
Spinach
Ginger (will help with the taste)

3. The Green Nutrient Juice

Kale
Watermelon

4. The Juice of your Dreams

Watermelon
Grapes
Pineapple
Strawberries
Spinach

5. The Extreme Health Juice

Kale
Garlic
Red Pepper
Tomato
Beets
Jalapeno

6. The Antioxidant Berry Juice

Red Grapes
Raspberries
Blueberries
Blackberries
Strawberries
One Lemon

7. Juice for Kids #1

Strawberries
1/2 Banana
Peach
Watermelon
Pineapple

8. Juice for Kids #2 *(add spinach if desired)*

Pineapple
1/2 Banana
Strawberries

9. Juice for Kids #3

Spinach
Watermelon
Pineapple

10. Juice for Kids #4

Orange
Banana
Strawberries

11. **Juice for Kids #5** *(add ice if desired)*

Lemons
Water
1 tsp. Agave

12. Juice for Kids #6 *(add spinach if desired)*

Peach

Strawberries
Mango

13. Reduce Inflammation #1

Apple
Strawberries
Lime

14. Reduce Inflammation #2

Apple
Pear
Carrot
Celery
Lemon
Turmeric Root
Ginger Root

15. Reduce Inflammation #3

Pineapple
Pear
Peach

16. Reduce Inflammation #4

Tomato
Celery
Cucumber
Carrot
Parsley
Spinach
Green Pepper

17. Reduce Inflammation #4

Apple
Pear
Celery
Orange
Sweet Potato

18. Reduce Inflammation #5

Carrot
Cucumber
Apple
Pear
Lemon
Spinach
Ginger Root

19. Reduce Inflammation #6

Blueberries
Strawberries
Kiwi
Peppermint

20. Reduce Inflammation #7

Tomato
Pepper
Celery
Cilantro
Onion
Garlic
Cayenne Pepper

21. Reduce Inflammation #8

Apple
Cucumber
Carrot
Grapes
Spinach
Green Pepper

22. The Stress Reliever Juice

Celery
Green Apples
Lemon
Handful of Spinach
Ginger Root

23. Kill That Headache Juice

Pineapple
Kale
Celery
Cucumber
Lemon
Ginger Root

24. The Energizer Juice

Tomatoes
Cucumber
Apples
Kale

25. The Cool-Me-Down Juice

Kiwi
Raspberries
Watermelon

26. The Grand Grapefruit Juice

Grapefruit
Orange
Carrot
Fresh Ginger

27. The Blueberry Lemon Juice

Spinach
Blueberries
Apple
Lemon

28. The Cool Cucumber Juice

Cucumber
Honeydew Melon
Lemon
Spinach
Mint

29. Mr. Mango Juice

Mango
Cucumber
Orange
Carrots

Spinach
Ginger

30. The Peaceful Peach Juice

Peaches
Banana
Lime

31. The Juice for Diabetics

Green Beans
Brussel Sprouts
Carrots
Beets

32. In Support of Breast Cancer

Watermelon
Strawberries
Raspberries
Pineapple

I'd like to add the following four recipes for those in need of a quick "get well," for those who are suffering from a cholesterol problem, a lack of potassium, calcium, or need to build up their blood.

1. The Blood Transfusion Juice

Carrot
Celery
Beet
Spinach
Kale
Red Bell Pepper

Ginger
Chard

2. The Calcium Rich Juice

Carrots
Dinosaur Kale
Parsley
1 Apple

3. The Anti-Cholesterol Juice

Parsley
Spinach
Garlic
Carrots
Small amount of Cayenne

4. The Potassium Juice

Celery
Spinach
Parsley
Carrots

Juicing Tip for Diabetics

Of all the vegetables that grow above ground, there are two in particular that are especially effective for diabetics. Green beans (aka string beans) and brussel sprouts. Both of these vegetables are unique in that they contain natural insulin, so making a juice that is a mixture of the two and drinking it daily is one of the best juicing recipes for diabetes.

When juicing, we want to focus more on vegetable juices rather than the fruit juice. We also want to focus on vegetables that are low in sugar content. As a general rule, vegetables that are grown above the ground are high in sugar. This includes beets, carrots, and yams. When starting juicing for the first time, I tell people to add a small amount of carrots to their juice to make the juices slightly more delicious. But the key here is a small amount. In time, you will want to remove the carrot from the drink and juice vegetables that have lower sugar content.

For those who don't have diabetes, I recommend that you continually learn and try new juice recipes. You should have a blast exploring the beautiful world of fruits and vegetables. Visit juice bars and check out their recipes. You'll see all types of mixtures for juices. I've given you 40 of my personal favorite recipes that I have tried and enjoyed. I've also personally experienced the benefits of these juice recipes. The good news is that you can mix them as you desire or need the certain benefit of each fruit or vegetable.

I'd have juice parties and invite family and friends over to try new juice combinations. It can be a lot of fun and a whole lot healthier than having a cook out or drinking all night. You would leave feeling healthy, clean and fresh. I personally host a lot of juicing parties, and they are a blast. In fact, I do a Healing and Weight Loss Retreat on St. Pete Beach and do juicing demonstrations all through my retreat. You owe it to yourself to attend at least one of my retreats before you die. You would leave forever changed and would have the most relaxing, fulfilling, life-changing and empowering 3 days of your life.

Chapter 8

Q & A's with Matt Maddix

In this chapter I'm going to answer the questions that I have received about juicing as well as health and weight loss. I'm going to be straightforward and transparent with each of my answers. I want to give you my heart on this and share with you why I am so passionate about juicing and health.

1. How much juice should I drink each day?

I recommend up to two 16-ounce glasses of fresh fruit juice and up two 24-ounce glasses of fresh vegetable juice a day for most people. I teach my clients in my weight loss coaching to drink at least two-four juices each day as a lifestyle.

2. Can I freeze or store the juices?

Yes. You will lose some of the nutritional benefits and enzymes, but it is better than letting the juice go to waste. However, I do recommend that you don't store in the refrigerator longer than 24 hours. It's always best and you'll get the most benefits to drink the juice right after you juice it.

3. What is the difference between a juicer and blender?

A juicer separates the liquid from the Fiber. A blender is designed to blend or liquefy food by chopping it up at high speeds. It doesn't separate the juice from the pulp, so the result is a mushy mess that really doesn't taste that good in some cases. Blenders can be quite useful. For example, bananas contain very little juice but taste delicious in drinks. The Nutri-Bullet is perfect because it liquefies the juice better than most blenders.

4. Is it ok to mix Fruits and Vegetables?

Sure you can. There is no set rule against mixing them. In fact some of the juicing combinations require for you to combine fruits with vegetables.

5. Do I have to follow the juice recipes exactly?

Absolutely not; juicing is meant to be fun. These recipes are only designed to point you in the right direction. Have a blast and create your own favorite combinations. Don't over-analyze the juicing experience. The more you juice, the more you will learn what combinations you prefer.

6. What is your favorite juice?

That is tough! I have a few favorites. My absolute favorite of all time is Carrot, Apple and Ginger. I also love Spinach, Watermelon, Pineapple and Grapes. I also love Kale, Tomatoes, Jalapeno, Red Pepper, Celery and Garlic. See, I told you it was tough. I just absolutely love juicing, period!

7. Should I only buy organic fruits and vegetables?

You should always buy organic fruits and vegetables if you can afford them. Organic produce also tends to yield more juice and have better flavor based on what's in season and where it's from. If you don't buy organic produce, I do recommend that you wash it thoroughly before juicing it. Here is a list of the fruits and vegetables that you must buy organic:

- *Apples*
- *Celery*
- *Cherry Tomatoes*

- *Cucumbers*
- *Grapes*
- *Hot Peppers*
- *Nectarines*
- *Peaches*
- *Potatoes*
- *Spinach*
- *Strawberries*
- *Bell Peppers*
- *Kale*
- *Summer Squash*
- *Raspberries*
- *Pears*
- *Blueberries*

If you must buy conventional, these are the safer choices:

- *Asparagus*
- *Broccoli*
- *Tomatoes*
- *Watermelon*
- *Avocados*
- *Cabbage*
- *Cantaloupe*
- *Sweet Corn*
- *Eggplant*
- *Grapefruit*
- *Kiwi*
- *Mangoes*
- *Mushrooms*
- *Onions*
- *Papayas*
- *Pineapples*
- *Sweet Peas*

- *Sweet Potatoes*
- *Lemons*
- *Bananas*

8. Why do I get Headaches while on a juice Fast?

This is perfectly normal during the first few days of juicing as your body is detoxifying. Stick with it, and you'll notice the headaches will disappear.

9. Where do you get protein on a juice fast?

You'll get plenty of protein from vegetables and fruits. You can find good protein in vegetables such as Spinach, Kale, Romaine Lettuce, Broccoli, Brussels Sprouts, Peas, Carrots, Turnip Greens and Collards.

10. Can I take my juice to work with me?

Of course you can. However, it's best to drink it fresh, so make and bring only the juices that you can't make and drink at home. Put your juice in a Mason jar and keep it cold in a cooler or the fridge. Make sure you drink the juice the day that you juice it. The Mayo Clinic says that it's essential to drink fresh juices as soon after they are made as possible because of their increased vulnerability to bacteria when stored.

11. Is it normal that my urine is a different color than normal when I juice?

Yes! You are ok. It's normal, and you have nothing to worry about. Since you are juicing mostly greens, your stool and urine will take on that color. It's the same if you juice a lot of beets. Keep on juicing, my friends.

12. What about the Sugar in the fruits; is it bad for you?

Unless you have blood sugar problems, there is no need for you to avoid fruit juices. The natural sugar in fruits is easily assimilated and digested, unlike white refined sugar, which is extremely harmful to the body. Fruits have a low glycemic index, which means that it doesn't make the glucose level in the blood rise as fast and high as white refined sugar or high fructose corn syrup. Sorry, you are not off the hook.

13. Should I wash all of my fruits and vegetables before juicing?

Yes! You should wash even if they are organic. Even organics have been sitting in trucks, handled by field hands and truckers. Run the fruit/vegetables under the water, this not only helps remove dirt and bacteria, but it also helps remove residual pesticides.

If you have some kind of brush to clean with, you may wish to use that for certain items, such as potatoes, lemons, apples, etc. Always wash your hands first before you handle the fruits and vegetables. Wait to wash right before you use the produce. Wash in a bowl of water and do not put the produce in the sink.

Some suggest mixing water with white vinegar and spraying on fruits/vegetables and leaving on for 30 seconds before rinsing them in water. Experts found that a white vinegar and water wash kills 98% of bacteria and removes pesticides. Please take this very seriously and always wash your fruits.

14. Why not just eat the fruits/vegetables rather than juice them?

It's best to juice your fruits and vegetables because most people don't consume enough to reap the benefits. Juicing is a much easier way to get the recommended amount of fruits and vegetables in your body. Both eating and juicing of your vegetables will give you essential nutrients needed by the body to help fight disease. If you can eat the same amount of fruits and vegetables that you would in juicing, by all means do it.

15. Can juicing replace meals?

Yes! However, remember that I recommend that you eat smaller portions at least 4-6 times a day. A glass of juice can be one of those 4-6 times. I do recommend that juicing becomes a part of your everyday lifestyle. I'd prefer that you treat juicing more like a snack rather than an actual meal.

16. Which types of Juicers are the best?

My personal favorite is the Nutri-Bullet and The Jack LaLanne. Juicers remove the pulp for easier digestion of juices, whereas blenders retain all parts of the fruits/vegetables and blend it up for a thicker drink. There are many juicers on the market. I also recommend, "The Health Master," "The Champion," and "The Vitamix!"

17. What if I hate the taste of juicing, and it grosses me out?

Suck it up! Stop psyching yourself out of juicing by allowing yourself to think about how "nasty" it is. Your thoughts, attitude and energy toward juicing will make a big difference in the experience. I see too many people who joke about it or talk about how "gross" it is before they even drink it.

However, I do suggest that you chug it down fast or even plug your noise if you have to. Whatever it takes to get it in your body, let's do it. Don't miss out on the health benefits of juicing because you "don't like it!" I do know that your taste buds will change and that your body will actually begin to crave it. The rewards of juicing far outweigh the "nasty" taste that you experience. Like I said from the beginning, "SUCK IT UP and JUST DO IT!" You will not regret being a daily juicer. However, I can promise you that if you continuously neglect your health and don't get serious about fruits and vegetables, you will end up with major regrets.

18. Do you eat meat? Is it ok to eat meat?

Yes I do eat meat, but very rarely. If I do have meat, I'm very focused on making sure that it is organic turkey, salmon, chicken or fish. Rarely do I ever eat red meat. I'm talking maybe about 4-6 times a year will I have a cheeseburger or steak. I've discovered that eating red meat is very unhealthy and puts you at risk of heart disease and cancer as well as other diseases. I'm going to strongly recommend that you eat meat in extreme moderation and be as careful as you are able to make sure that it's organic meat.

19. Why do you think that Dairy is bad for you?

I rarely eat any dairy cheeses and never drink dairy milk. I've switched over to goat cheese and almond milk. Contrary to popular belief, eating dairy products has never been shown to reduce fracture risk. In fact, some studies indicate that it increases it as much as by 50 percent. Dairy is linked to one of the primary causes of prostrate cancer and heart disease. Dairy causes digestive problems and aggravates irritable bowel syndrome. Dairy also contributes to more health problems such as: allergies, sinus problems, ear infections, type 1 diabetes and headaches.

There is no cholesterol or saturated fat in almond milk. It's low in sodium and high in healthy fats such as omega fatty acids, typically found in fish, which help to prevent high blood pressure and heart disease. Almond milk (with no additives) is low in carbs, which means it won't significantly increase your blood sugar levels, thus reducing your risk for diabetes. Almond milk is high in vitamins and minerals. I always get the unsweetened Almond Milk. My son actually loves it more than Dairy milk. You'll never want to go back to Dairy when you stop eating and drinking it. I've reduced all inflammation in my bad knee after cutting out dairy. I can run 10 miles with no pain and before, I couldn't even run around the block.

20. How much Fiber is too much Fiber?

The national fiber recommendations are 30-38 grams a day for men and 25 grams a day for women between 18 and 50 years old. Most Americans get less than 15 grams of fiber per day. Spread out your fiber intake throughout the day. This is why I suggest eating small portions every 2-3 hours each day. Make sure that you drink a lot of water. The more fiber that you eat, the more fluid that your body needs. Just be cautious not to overdo anything when it comes to your body.

21. What kind of Protein Shake do you drink?

I drink Organic Whey Protein with Almond Milk and Peanut Butter about twice per day. Usually one in the morning and one right after I work out. I pour the Almond Milk in the Nutri-Bullet, put two scoops of Whey Protein and a scoop of Peanut Butter, and it's absolutely delicious.

22. What if my family won't support my juicing lifestyle?

Keep a positive attitude about it, but don't let their negative words or attitude keep you from doing what you know is right for your health. Set the example and let them see the results from juicing. Have a meeting with your family and ask for their support. Be very clear that your intention is not to push your passion on them but that you would like for them to try different juices until they find ones they like. If you have a spouse that is overweight or trying to get healthy, make sure that you give them 100% support and do the journey with them.

23. Should I remove the seeds from the Apple before juicing them?

Yes you should. It takes just a little bit longer but wise to remove them. However, do not panic if you should put them through the Jack LaLane juicer. It will not have an effect on you at all. Apple seeds are extremely poisonous and could kill you if you eat enough of them. Just to be safe, I cut my apples so that the seeds never go in my juices.

24. Is it ok to drink juices in stores that say, "100% Juice"?

Absolutely not! There is nothing that replaces raw vegetable or fruit juice at home with your own juicer. So what does 100% juice on the label mean? Not much at all. Food companies are allowed to say 100% juice on the label even though their juice contains additional additives, flavorings and preservatives. The word "concentrate" is just a fancy name for syrup. Juice concentrates are made from vegetables and fruits that are heated down to syrup and then have water added back in. The concentration process involves both adding in and subtracting chemicals and natural plant products in order to condense the juice.

Many juice companies use an ingredient called citric acid to extend the shelf life of their product. Most would think that citric acid comes from citrus lemons, oranges and limes, but it doesn't. The ingredients most of these companies use to create citric acid are genetically engineered sugar beets. There is nothing "healthy" about store bought orange, apple or grape juice. Go for the authentic real and healthy and make your own juice.

25. Are Naked Juice Drinks Good for you?

NO! Of course they might be better than a Coke or Mountain Dew. However, they are not healthy at all. Again, make your own juice and drink water. You are much better off without all the other store bought junk. Naked was recently sued because they claimed their juices were 100% all natural but really were hiding GMO and synthetic ingredients, including zinc oxide, ascorbic acid, and calcium pantothenate, which is produced from formaldehyde.

This example is just one of the reasons why it's so important that you always look at the ingredient list first rather than trusting labels that say, "All Natural!" If you are unable to make your own juice for whatever reason, make sure that you choose organic juice first and foremost. So if you are going to buy juice from the store, make sure that it's organic and cold pressed.

If you have other questions that I can answer for you, I do a LIVE Daily Internet Talk Show every Monday at 9 am about Health and Weight Loss. Join us at fuelforsuccess.tv to watch live, and you can also watch any of our previous 200 Episodes in the archives. My partner, Mike Hopkins, and I do a 30-minute Health Show every Monday and would love to help you with any additional questions.

Chapter 9

How to Raise Healthy Kids

I do not speak to you in this chapter as someone who is giving advice on something that I personally haven't had to live out in the trenches. I'm a very busy single dad who has a very demanding schedule and still somehow am able to motivate my 12-year-old son (Caleb) to eat healthy and love juicing.

We as parents can't afford to wait until they are teenagers to try to teach them how to be healthy. It's our responsibility to prepare our kids for adulthood. Our sweet little children are learning habits and behavior patterns that are going to stick with them when are they are adults. Think of the challenge that we currently face in changing our habits and behaviors as adults. We as parents can make it easier on our children by teaching them while they are young how to develop daily habits for healthy eating and living a healthy life.

There are approximately 13 million obese children in America who struggle with obesity. Personally I hold the parents responsible for allowing their children to develop bad habits. I've watched so many parents actually condition their children to become emotional eaters. We take them out for Ice Cream after the Dr. visits or after their arm is broken as a way to make them feel better. We are condoning their desire for bad foods when bad things happen or when they are feeling emotionally low. Don't get me wrong, I'm okay with giving our kids Ice Cream, but I don't believe we should use foods as a way of consoling their emotions. For example, one day Caleb and I were watching a movie at home, and I had been noticing that every time we watched a movie, he would want a "snack." We could have just had dinner 30 minutes prior, yet he would ask for a snack even though he wasn't actually hungry. Therefore, one night I said, "Caleb no more snacking during movies unless it's fruit or vegetables; if you are not careful you are going to train your brain and body to need food every time that you watch a movie." It's okay to enjoy a healthy snack when you watch a movie, but I just didn't want it to become habitual or physiological for him. I was doing my job as a parent by teaching him to control any type of emotional eating and helping him to develop the right habits. Thankfully, whenever we watch a movie now, he says, "Dad can you make a plate of fresh fruit?" I'd much rather that he request fresh fruit than Nacho's, Pizza, or any other junk food. His brain is now trained.

I'm going to give you 5 tips for motivating and training your kids to live a healthy lifestyle.

1. **Start while they are young.**

   Far too many parents wait until their children become teenagers before they teach them the right habits. We must start teaching them healthy habits as young as possible if we want our children to live a healthy lifestyle. I've watched the power of starting young with my own son. He is only 12 years old and already lives a healthier lifestyle than most adults that I know. The reason for my success in training my son to enjoy juicing and exercise is because I started really young with him.

   Remember that eating a healthy lifestyle is not a punishment or a drag. Living a lifestyle of juicing, exercise and healthy eating is a blessing. Therefore, don't feel guilty as a parent because you are teaching your children at a young age to juice and eat healthy. I've had other parents give me the strangest looks when I said that Caleb was not allowed to drink Coke. It's my choice as a parent and when he is older, he can make that choice to drink Coke if he so desires. However, I've never given him permission to order a Coke because it's so bad for you, and I want his body to crave water and fresh juice. I've tested this by letting him order a Coke, and he wasn't even able to finish it. His body rejected it because it was used to water and juice only. One of the best pieces of advice that I could give anyone when it comes to health and juicing is to realize that what you put into your body, your body will begin to crave.

2. **Model a Healthy Lifestyle.**

If we really want to make a huge impact on the health of our children, we must lead by example by showing them what living a healthy lifestyle looks like. Our children are like sponges; they soak up everything that they see and hear from us. My son told me that he doesn't remember a day in his life where he hasn't heard the sound of a juicer in the kitchen. I'm so grateful that he has the sounds of a juicer that deep in his subconscious mind. I've modeled a lifestyle of daily juicing before him, and he knows by my example that I take our health very seriously.

You can start by making healthy choices when you are at a restaurant and showing them how to look at the menu carefully and ask key questions to the server about how much sugar or salt is used. Is the Salmon wild caught or farm raised? Asking these types of questions in front of our children will show them by example to slow down and carefully consider what they are about to order. I'll even ask the server, "What are the top 3 Healthiest things on the menu?" Caleb has watched me do that so much that now even at the age of 12 he is starting to ask the same thing.

Just like anyone else, my son loves his sweets. However, he knows that as a lifestyle, we only eat sweets once a week. I'm very calculated with this habit. It's part of our lifestyle. As a lifestyle, we get one cheat day! The other 6 days we stay very consistent with our juicing and clean eating lifestyle. Parents, don't be aimless when it comes to food. We need to have a plan and show our kids the value of planning their meals and picking the day that will be their cheat day. Having a cheat day is okay in moderation.

Or course my son loves his Chic-Fil-A and would eat it everyday if I were to allow him. Even though I am a fan of Chic-Fil-A, I only let him eat this once a week as well. Remember, we can't be careless about our health. We have to have habits and discipline. Too many people just eat fast food, pizza, burgers and sweets whenever, and most don't even truly know how many times a week they are eating it.

3. Don't buy junk and bring it home.

Too many kids have entirely too much access to unhealthy foods right at home. Caleb often laughs at me when he comes to my house because he literally only sees fresh fruits, vegetables, nuts and teas. Too many people snack on junk food, chips, etc. because they have quick access to it in their cupboards. Friends, if you want to live a healthy lifestyle, fill your refrigerator and pantry with healthy organic foods as much as possible. Trust me on this; if you don't have the sweets at home, the Cokes or the junk food, you'll not be as tempted to eat it. I tell all of my clients that I do Health Coaching for to go home and have a throw-it-away or give-it-away party by removing everything from their house that is bad for them by throwing it away or giving it away. This works and has a way of increasing energy, confidence and momentum toward their new healthy lifestyle. You will feel power over unhealthy food the day that you get rid of it and then decide to never bring it in your home again.

4. Make physical exercise part of your daily routine.

Caleb will tell you that I'm very strict about him doing his daily walk/jog. It's important to me that he does it on a daily basis. I've set a goal for him to do at least 20 minutes of cardio each day. It must be 20 straight minutes for the purpose of exercise. I know a lot people who say, "I walk from my car to work; is it okay to count that?" No! It's not okay. We all need actual time for exercise on a daily basis. Again, it's all about habits and lifestyle. This is why I make sure that he does 20 minutes everyday.

By my son doing 20 minutes of walking, swimming, jogging or biking each day, he is conditioning his mind and body to commit to daily exercise for the rest of his life. It literally has become second nature to where he does his 20 minutes of cardio daily without any need for a push or motivation. If we want healthy kids, we must make exercise part of their daily routine. This is not an option if we are serious about health. Too many children are growing up in homes where there is no physical exercise exampled to them and this is one of the reasons why childhood obesity is out of control in America.

5. Teach your children to love nature.

Just last night I took Caleb down to the beach at Sunset for a walk and jog. It was so beautiful, refreshing and cleansing. It's so important for our children to fall in love with nature. God created such a beautiful world and being out in nature is a way to connect with God and have your spiritual batteries recharged.

I can see such a difference in Caleb's energy and attitude after a long hike in the woods or a walk down the beach. Being outside in nature is so important for the wellness and health of our children. Too many children these days are stuck inside, glued to video games and are missing out on the beauty and blessing of nature. We grew up in a world where we played outside all day. This video game generation knows almost nothing of what this is like. It seems that parks are empty and most children are all inside playing video games. This is another cause of childhood obesity.

As parents, we need to take our kids for hikes, walks, bike rides, to parks, the beach, the mountains and the woods. We need more canoe rides, camping trips, walks in the forest, fishing, hunting, roller blading, bike riding, running, hammocks, picnics and just simply sitting by the fire at night watching the stars. Our children are growing up and almost completely losing touch with the beauty and healing of nature. Parents, please give your children the gift of being out in God's beautiful nature more.

Healthy Ideas for Children:

- *Juice everyday*
- *Exercise everyday*
- *Drink water with lemon*
- *Eat oatmeal in the morning*
- *Eat Fruit for Snacks*
- *Play outside*
- *Walk 20 minutes each day*

- *Go on hikes*
- *Go for bike rides*
- *Vacation in a Cabin in the mountains*
- *Walk the beach*
- *Go swimming*
- *Go out on the boat*
- *Lay in the hammock*
- *Take a picnic*
- *Go canoeing*
- *Go camping*
- *Eat more Salads*
- *Eat Wild Caught Salmon*
- *Eat Broccoli*
- *Laugh and Have Fun*

These are just a few things that we can do with our children. Parents, take this seriously and really give your kids the gift of a healthy lifestyle. Make it easier on them as adults by giving them the right healthy habits while they are young. You only get 18 short years until they are considered an adult. We have to be focused as parents and really do our jobs well. We can't get so caught up with life that we forget to play with our kids, laugh together and live life to the fullest. I'm determined that my son is going to see a happy, healthy and fun father. We have a blast together! We enjoy making many memories out in nature and have so much fun juicing and learning about health together. Don't be afraid to tell your kids, "No!" They will test you. However, you are the parent and you must love your children enough to give them a lifestyle of health and wellness. They will thank you for this one-day down the road when they are old enough to understand.

While some might consider me to be a little extreme, the result is that my son doesn't have to deal with obesity or the negative side effects of eating junk food. Remember, if you eat right, you will feel right. Many of Caleb's teachers, friends and coaches all comment on how much energy that Caleb seems to always have. Usually I just smile and say, "Thank you!" However, sometimes I'll break out a little speech about juicing, exercise and eating right and how much those 3 things can completely renew massive energy in our bodies. Parents, give your children a lifestyle of happiness, abundance, energy, wellness and health by teaching them to juice and exercise everyday of their life. You'll never regret this for one minute of your life. You will be so grateful that you taught your children how to have healthy habits. They will not struggle as much when they are adults and will have more personal discipline than most of their peers and co-workers in every other area of their life. I've learned that when we conquer the food demons, every other area of our life is impacted as well.

Chapter 10

If I Had My Life To Live Over Again

It has been a beautiful Friday in the state of Florida and in my life. I awoke early this morning to finish my "Must Be Done List" and accomplish my daily goals. I was able to make it to the gym for a workout and the downtown St. Pete for a run at sunrise on the water.

After swinging by the health food store to get my daily wheat grass shot, I decided to visit one of my favorite hangout spots in St. Petersburg - Mazzaros! If you are ever in the St. Petersburg area and want to have the experience of your life, then stop by Mazzaros. The place is electrifying with its Italian music, culture, and atmosphere. The coffee bar in the middle is my favorite spot to hang out, write and socialize with people. Everyone in that place knows me and treats me like a celebrity when I walk in. It's fun and very energizing to talk, laugh, and connect with all the workers.

Today, a very cute, elderly couple sitting right next to me caught my attention, and I decided to question them about life, family, success and passion. I enjoy talking with people and thoroughly believe that I can learn something from everyone that I meet. It is said that experience is the best teacher, but I'll have to disagree. Experience alone isn't the best teacher. The best teacher is your personal experience combined with the experience of others. During my enlightening, hour-long conversation with the 79-year-old couple, I learned that they had been married for 60 years. Their zest for life left me feeling refreshed, enriched, and thankful for my own life. I also was left with the feeling that life really does go by way too fast.

Later, while reminiscing with my brother Joe about this encounter, I became very sober when I related my final question to the elderly gentlemen and heard his response. I had said, "Jim, if you had it to do over again, what would you do differently?" He looked right into my eyes and said, "I'd do what I really wanted to do!" Then he said, "Matt, sadly I don't get to do it over again!"

For the past hour, I've been thinking about that one sentence. I'm in deep thought right now, there is a lump in my throat, and I have even been choked up a few times over the past few minutes. What would we all do if we had it to do over again? It's a fun question to ask everyone that we meet, but the fact of the matter is that we will never have an opportunity to live life over again. It is very sobering to remember that "We all have only ONE life!" One chance to do it!

We have one shot and one chance to learn our lessons, make our mark and experience life. No doubt there'll come a day that you'll look back, and it will be too late to live your dreams and passions. Someone once said, "When we get to the end of our lives, we'll not regret the things that we did, but rather the things that we didn't do!" So, what is it that you really want? What would you do with your life if you could have the "perfect" life? What would you do if you had to do it over again? What would you do if money was not an option and you could actually have the confidence to try and do what your heart beats for? What do you daydream about? What is burning in your soul and mind to do? What if you knew that it was impossible for you to fail? I urge you to stop right now and make sure you are living the life of your dreams now. Look within and turn a deaf ear to those small-minded critics who are always dragging you down with their average and mediocre words and thoughts. Please don't get to the end and regret. Please don't die with your dream inside! Please don't allow the fear of the unknown to keep you from living your life to the fullest. You have what it takes! God didn't put you on this earth for you to give in to your fears and settle for less than what you were born to do.

Anyone who studies success knows that "clarity" is the secret to achieving and getting what you want. Are you able to "clarify" exactly what you want, and then are you willing to pursue it regardless of the price you must pay to get it? Why don't you go back to school? Why not take that missions trip? Why not take your parents on their "dream" vacation? Why not build that Homeless Shelter? Why don't you quit that job that you hate and start your own business? Follow your passion! Yes! Go for it and don't look back. Burn the ships and decide that you are going to live everyday of your life doing what you love. Why don't you save the money and take your family on that vacation? Why not slow down and go play catch with your son, have that talk with your daughter, or go play games with your friends? Wake up everyday with purpose and passion! Go get what you deserve. Love yourself more and stop selling yourself so short in life.

I'm bothered with how stressed and unhappy America has become. We seem to be in such a hurry, rushing and going nonstop. We are living in fear of rejection and have settled with schedules we don't like while working jobs that we hate. What? You are going to give 40 hours of your week away, doing what you have no passion for? Why? For what? Security, a car you don't like, and a house you don't really enjoy? Why not make some radical changes? Change your spending habits, get out of debt, and do what you must do to start doing what you love and what you want. Are you willing to break out of your rut and take a leap or risk? I always like to operate with the worst case scenario in mind: what is the worst thing that could happen? If necessary, you become the biggest penny-pinching miser, get rid of the car payment, and live below your means until you are able to do what you love. It's a mind-over matter decision for seeing the big picture of your dreams and passions. If necessary, sell everything that you have and live in your car. Basically, you must be willing to literally do whatever it takes. You may have to work two jobs for just one year, get up at 4:00 am to study and read. You may have to say "no" to the good so you can say "yes" and enjoy the best. Whatever you do, please don't fall into the trap of selling yourself short. Please don't allow your father's negative opinion, your ex-husband, your friends, or even your past to keep you from a bright, healthy, exciting, passionate, and successful future. Your future is right now, and I want you to get off "Someday Island!" You say, "Someday I'll..." I'll what? How about doing it now and enjoying your life today? How about playing with your kid now? How about reading that book this week? How about joining the gym and making up your mind that you are going to walk right in there and work that fat right off your body? How about calling your dad now? How about inviting the family over this Sunday for dinner? How about less negativity, less TV time and more play time? How about going to the mall and buying yourself that dress that you really want?

Please slow down and get out of the boring, monotonous, and dissatisfying rut; live it up. Please dream and think as big as you possibly can. Please wake up with fresh passion tomorrow and live life to the fullest. Please do something for yourself. Please enjoy, laugh and love! Please give to your family and to others. Please don't make your wife read a romance novel to discover romance and passion. Please don't make your kids wonder what you were like! Please be with them, and when you are with your family, be with your family mentally, physically, and emotionally. Don't make your family attend your funeral before you were supposed to die! Don't make your kids grow up without a dad because you neglected your health. I can't even tell you how many frustrating funerals that I have been to because the person really didn't have to die. Even as I write this chapter today, I got the sad news of a young man in his 30's, a father of 4 who died today. It makes me angry because he didn't have to die. He was massively obese and sadly lost his life today and left his children behind to live the rest of their life without their daddy.

I've met hundreds of people in hospital beds who faced major regret that they didn't take better care of their health. Sometimes it's a wake-up call, causing many to make the necessary changes in their health so they can now live healthy and radiant lives. However, there are many of them who faced the reality that it was too late to exercise, juice and eat healthy. It's so alarming to me to think that all people had to do was juice, eat healthier and exercise on a consistent basis and they wouldn't have gotten diabetes, heart disease or cancer. I realize there are rare cases when sickness and disease strikes those who eat right, exercise and juice. However, it's extremely rare that sickness and disease hits those who live a healthy lifestyle. Friends, life is too short to waste our days away in sickness or in hospitals. I am a fanatic and radical about juicing and health because I love life so much and I want to live as long as I possibly can. However, not only do I want to live a long life, I also want to live life with the highest amount of energy, passion, wellness and health. Not only does juicing keep us from sickness, but it also gives us a better quality of life. Juicing and physical exercise will help you sleep better, feel better and live with the highest level of energy possible.

Whatever you do, please let this book serve as your wake-up call. Don't wait until it's too late before you decide to get healthy. Regardless of how bad you've neglected your health, don't stay in that rut and continue to abuse your health. Believe me, the pain of discipline is far less than the pain of regret. Many people have said to me, "I can't afford to juice!" Friends, you can't afford not to juice! The cost of medications, doctor's visits and being in the hospital will cost you much more than you've ever thought about spending on juicing and health.

Thank you so much for taking the time to read this book. I'm so grateful that you care enough about your health and your family to learn about health and wellness. You can do this! I know beyond a shadow of a doubt that you can get healthy, lose weight and find healing from sickness and disease through juicing and exercise. If I can help you in any way, please visit my website at mattmaddix.com. I'd be honored to be your personal life or health coach. Here are 5 reasons why my coaching will benefit you:

1. Healthy Lifestyle

I'm extremely focused on helping you develop a Healthy Lifestyle that will change your eating habits. This will not only help you lose weight; you'll also become a Healthier person! A healthier you will have more energy, be more focused and determined to reach your goal. I'm going to teach you how to make healthy choices to retrain your mind and body to want to be Healthy! Quick weight loss is not the way to go because the weight loss doesn't last and you become discouraged. I truly believe that establishing correct habits is the secret to a healthy lifestyle. My method is practical, achievable and simple. I'm with you every step of the way!

2. Meal Planning

Most people don't live a healthy life because they don't have a plan. "Failure to plan is planning to fail!" I will show you How to plan your meals, exercise and start juicing with foods you enjoy. Planning will give you confidence that you CAN succeed!

3. Extreme Motivation

I have the ability to motivate people to become self-motivated and focus on doing whatever it takes. People who use my coaching program reach their weight loss goal because of the encouragement and motivation I bring to their lives. I will motivate you to live a healthy life, make healthy choices and start transforming your life!

4. Accountability

The most valuable part of my process is the interactive accountability! One reason people don't change is because they are not accountable to anyone. Not only will our weekly coaching sessions help with this, but you will also text me throughout the process. You will text me after each meal you eat and after you complete your daily exercise. This will help you think twice about reaching for that unhealthy food! My previous clients have found this to be the key in helping them break through in their weight loss process.

5. Success and Results

Friend, the major benefit of having me as your weight loss coach is that I produce results 100% of the time! This process will help you live with maximum energy, confidence, and health. I will help you learn how to release all negative emotions and energy! You will become emotionally and mentally strong to overcome food addiction, emotional eating, and change your life habits! Say good-bye to low self-esteem, rejection, unworthiness and depression! I'm going to help you Love yourself! Get ready to come alive, become stronger, healthier and more confident than you have EVER been! You WILL lose the weight and learn to become a very healthy person!

What's stopping you from daily exercise, consistent juicing and living a healthy lifestyle? Since we don't have it to do over again, why not do it now?

Author Bio

Matt Maddix is a highly sought after Motivational Speaker and Life Coach. As the CEO and Founder of Matt Maddix Motivations, Matt has authored 5 Books and has hosted over 100 live training events; motivating and training over 32,000 registered attendees.

Matt is also the Co-Founder of Mission 25, a Missions Movement in America and Daily Internet Talk Show "Fuel for Success!" Matt Maddix has traveled across the world for the past 15 years doing over 2,000 live speaking events to audiences as large as 15,000 people.

Matt is an expert in motivation, life coaching, sales training, relationships, success, entrepreneurship and business growth. He is also one the most effective Weight Loss Coaches in the world.

Matt Maddix resides in the Tampa Bay area with his son Caleb.

Matt is available for speaking engagements, weight loss coaching and life coaching. For additional information, visit his website at: mattmaddix.com.